Contents

Preface to the third edition

Six years have elapsed since the publication of the second edition of this book. This new edition has undergone major changes. The questions are arranged in a random fashion and not according to specific categories and are also more diverse in order to make them more interesting to the reader. Many new illustrations have been added and the number of page spreads has been increased from 50 to 100 making a total of 200 questions. The main aim of this book, however, remains unchanged: to enhance the reader's ability to remember facts about many ophthalmic conditions.

JJK

Acknowledgements

I am very grateful to Aasheet Desai for his advice and suggestions. I am also extremely grateful to the following colleagues and medical photographers for providing images. I. Gout, C. Barry, K. Sehmi, P. Saine, R. Curtis, S. Milewski, L. Merin, P. Gilli, U. Kaul Raina, L. MacKeen, A. Pearson, R. Marsh, A. Curi, N. Byer, P. Watson, C. Pavesio, S. Tuft, J. Harry, J. Sloper, A. McIntyre, V. Tanner, B. Damato, N. Sibtain, K. Nischal, D. Taylor, J. Salmon, H. Mroczkowska, N. Raik, N. Rogers, S. Fogla, R. Visser, W. Lisch, L. Horton, R. Chopdar, A. Garner, S. Delva, S. Webber, G. Rose, S. Kumar Puri, J. Yanguela, D. Armstrong, J. Dart, G. Misson, M. Kerr-Muir, R. Packard, S. Mitchell, S. Lightman, A. Moore, T. ffytche, A. Singh, M. Hamza, S. S. Hayreh, P. Watts, J. Govan, K. Jordan, M. Parulekar, D. Thomas, E. Pringle, M. A. Mir, and C. Gilbert.

Section 1

Questions 1 to 50. Answers start on page 52.

Q 1 Match 1 with one of (A–D)

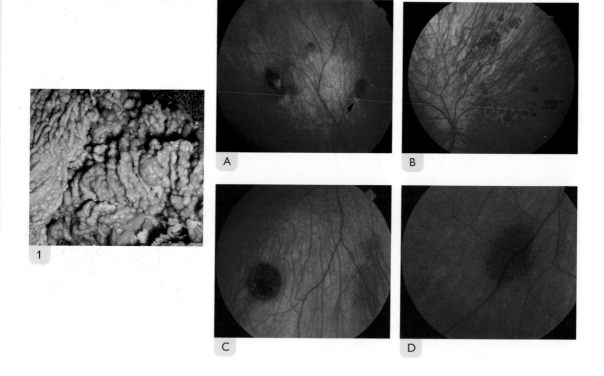

Answer on page 52

Q 2 Match the fundus (1–3) with the CT (A–C)

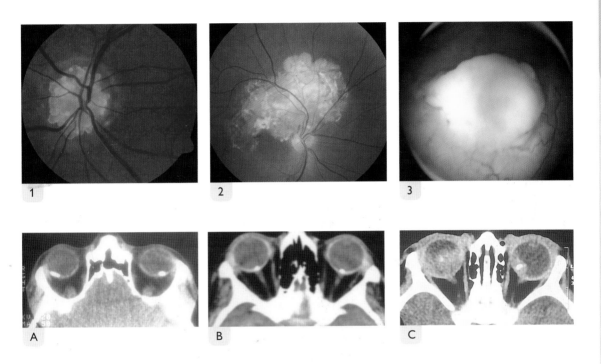

Answer on pages 52–53

Q 3 What do these fluorescein angiograms show?

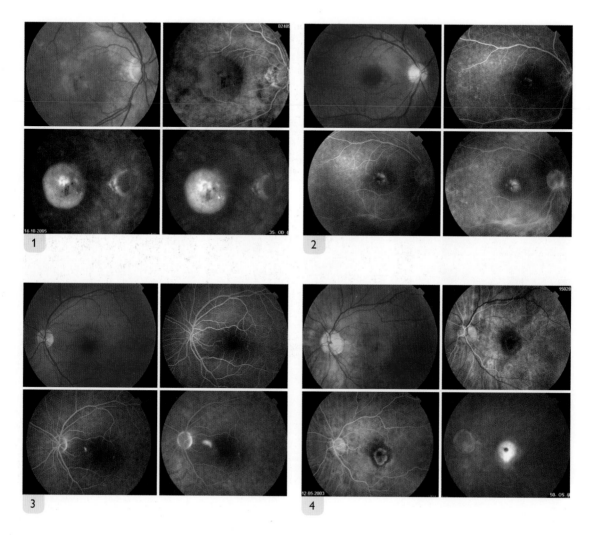

Answer on page 53

Q 4 Herpes simplex or herpes zoster?

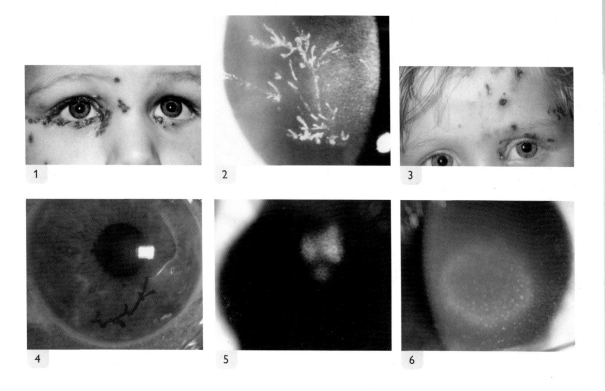

1

2

3

4

5

6

Answer on pages 53–54

Q **5** Two systemic diseases are shown: match each ocular sign (1 and 2) with the systemic feature (A–D)

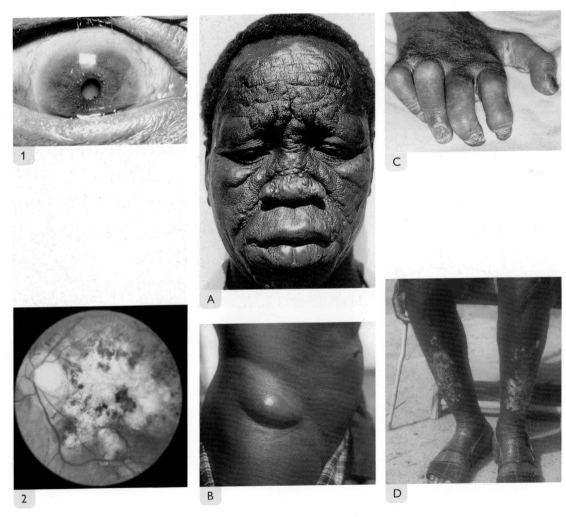

Answer on page 54

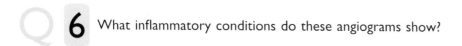

Q 6 What inflammatory conditions do these angiograms show?

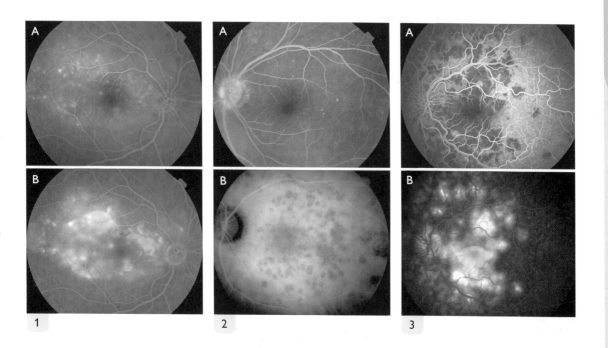

A

B

1

A

B

2

A

B

3

Answer on page 55

Q 7 Match the uveitis (1–3) with the pathogen (A–C)

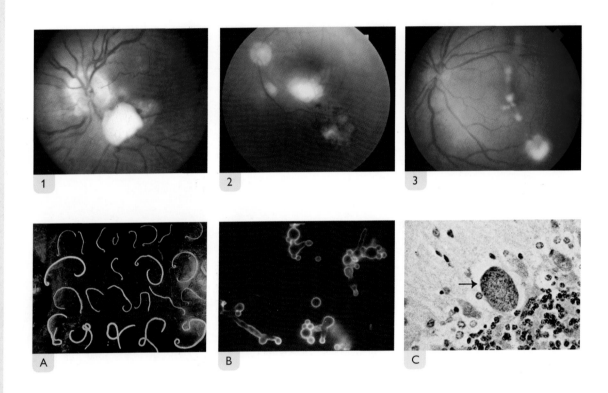

Answer on pages 55–56

Q 8 Match the keratic precipitates (1–3) with (A–C)

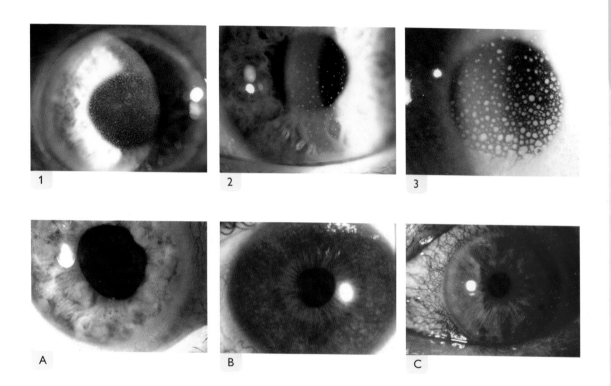

Answer on page 56

Q 9 Match the hands (1–3) with the eye (A–C)

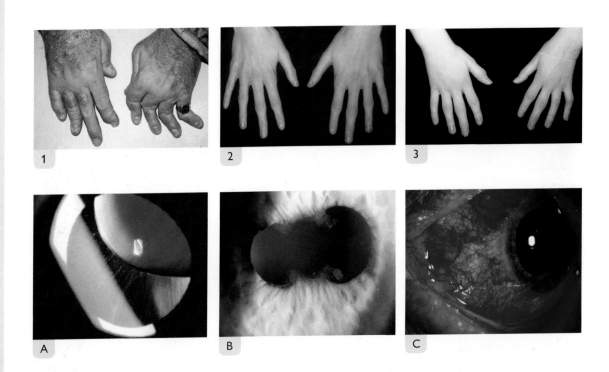

Answer on pages 56–57

Q 10 Match the face (1–3) with the iris (A–C)

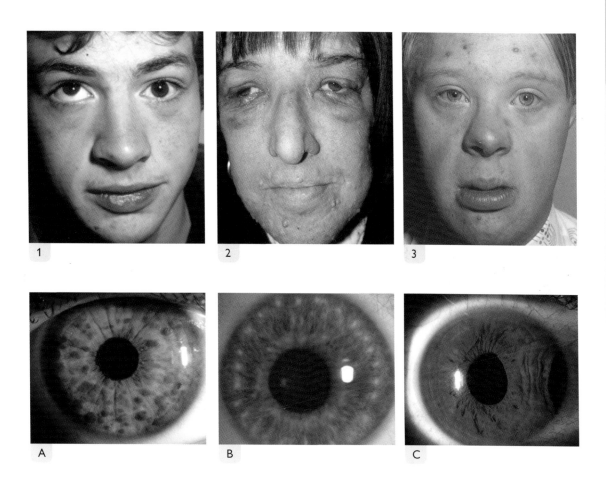

Answer on page 57

Q 11   What are the wild animal connotations?

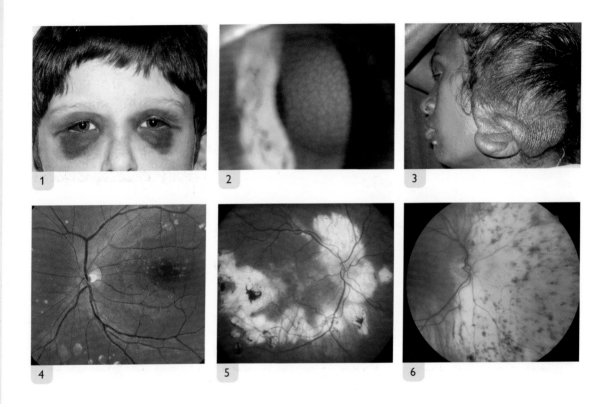

1

2

3

4

5

6

Answer on pages 57–58

Q 12 What are the animal connotations?

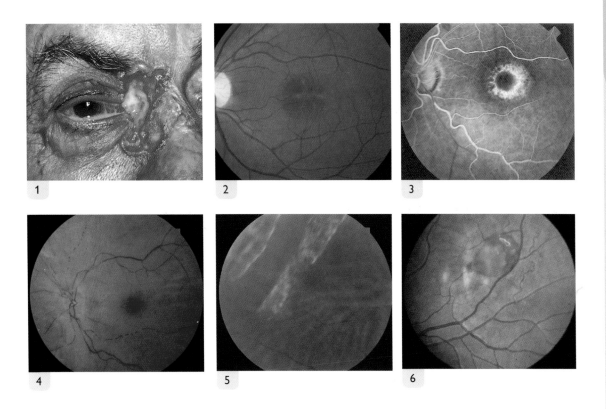

1

2

3

4

5

6

Answer on page 58

Q **13** Which of these are not associated with recurrent corneal erosions?

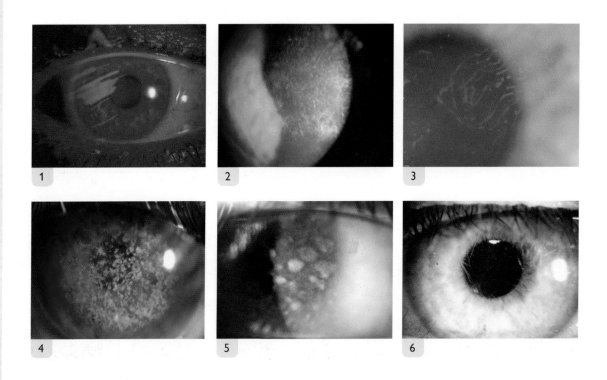

Answer on pages 58–59

Q 14 What is the probable associated refraction?

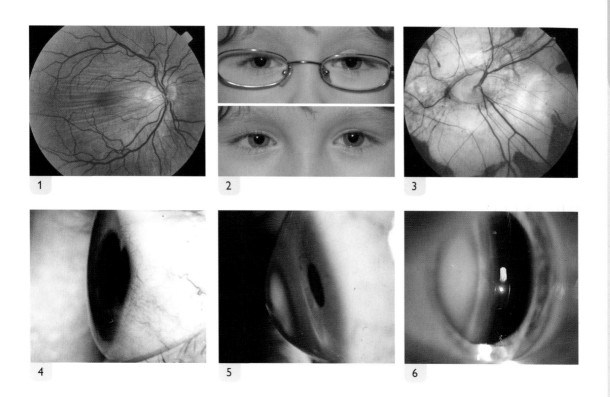

1

2

3

4

5

6

Answer on pages 59–60

Q 15 What is this condition?

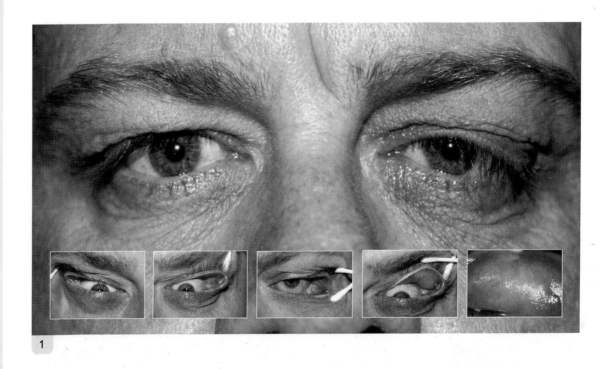

1

Answer on page 60

Q **16** Match the face (1–3) with the cataract (A–C)

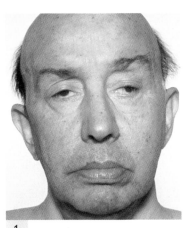

1

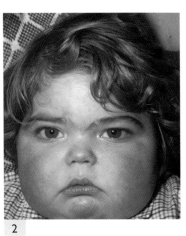

2

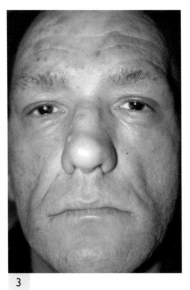

3

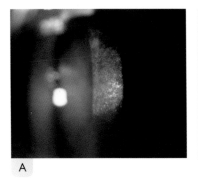

A

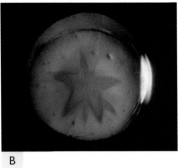

B

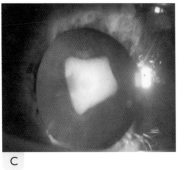

C

Answer on pages 60–61

Q 17 Match the drug side effect (1–3) with the indication for its use (A–C)

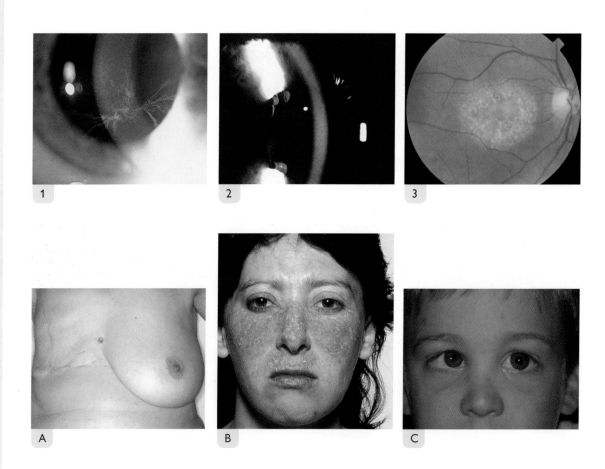

Answer on page 61

Q 18 Match the fundus dystrophy (1–3) with the findings in carriers (A–C)

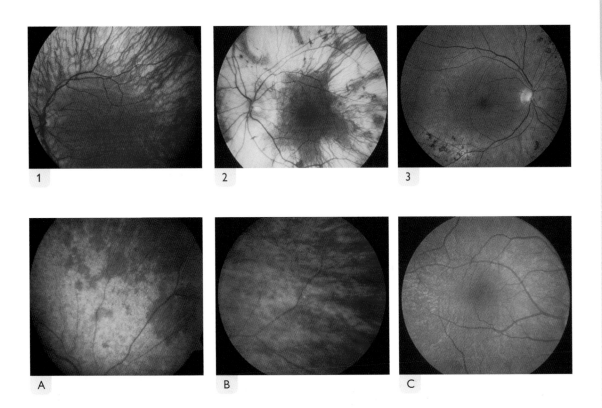

1

2

3

A

B

C

Answer on pages 61–62

Q 19 Match the eyelid lesion (1–3) with the histology (A–C)

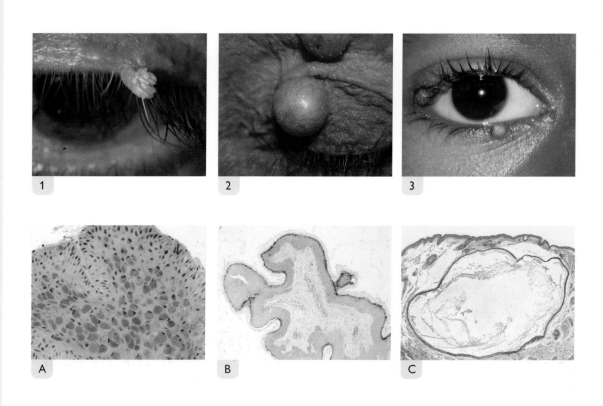

Answer on page 62

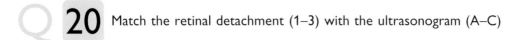

Q 20 Match the retinal detachment (1–3) with the ultrasonogram (A–C)

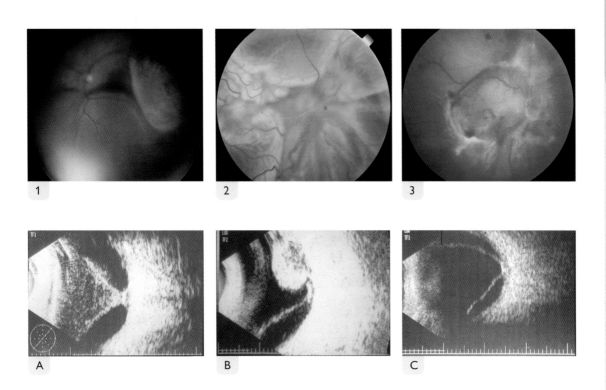

Answer on pages 62–63

Q 21 Match (1–3) with the gonioscopy (A–C)

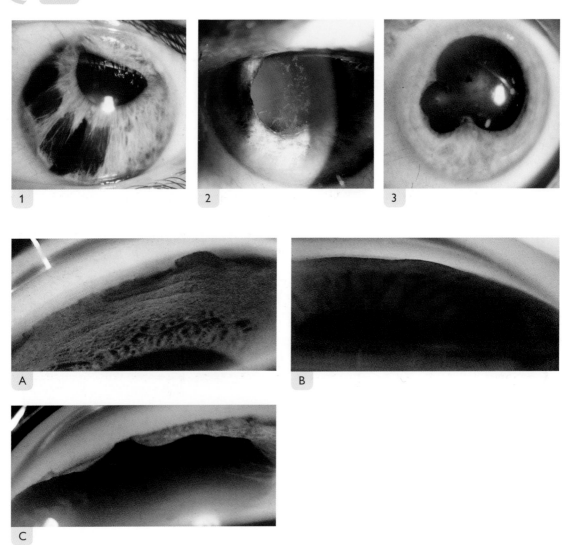

Answer on page 63

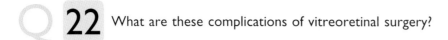

Q 22 What are these complications of vitreoretinal surgery?

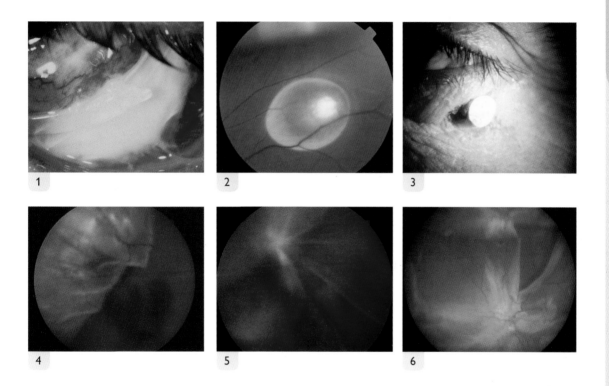

1

2

3

4

5

6

Answer on page 63

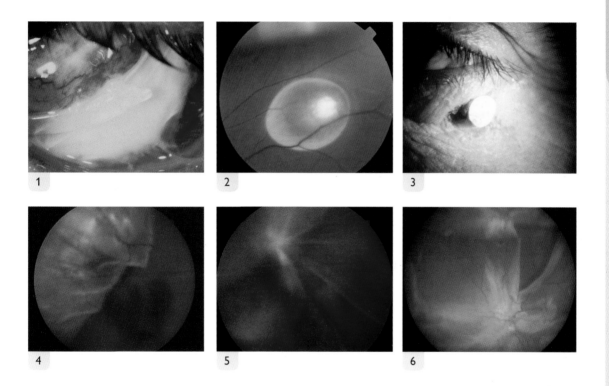

Q 23 What have these conditions in common?

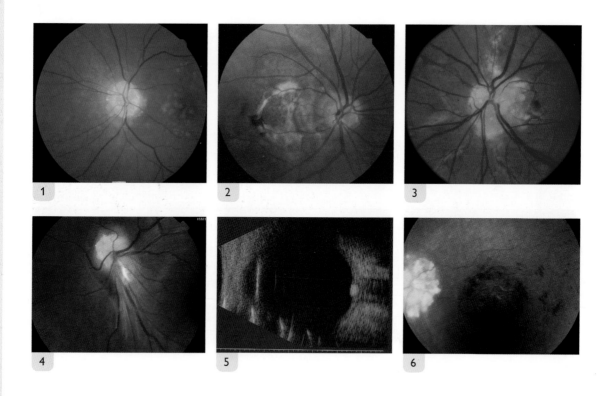

Answer on page 64

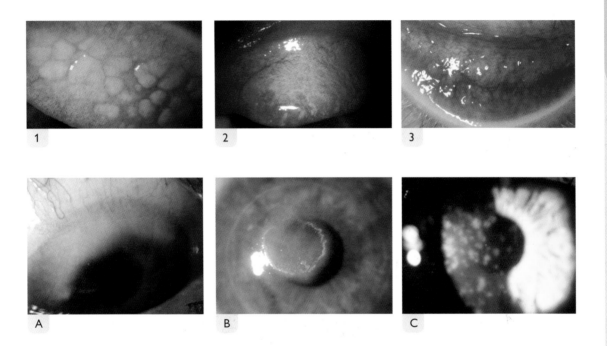

1

2

3

A

B

C

Answer on page 64

Q 25 Match the blepharitis (1–3) with the dermatitis (A–C)

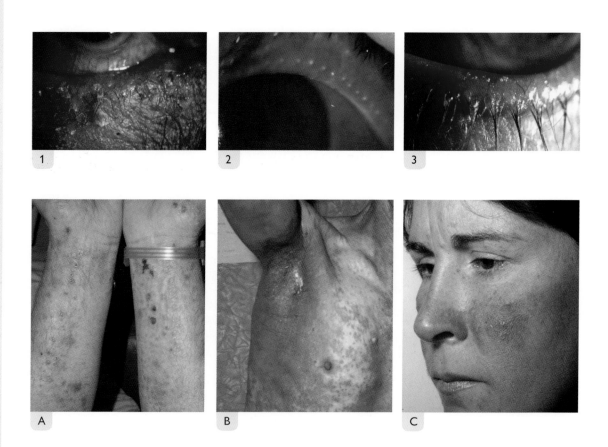

Answer on page 65

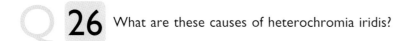

Q **26** What are these causes of heterochromia iridis?

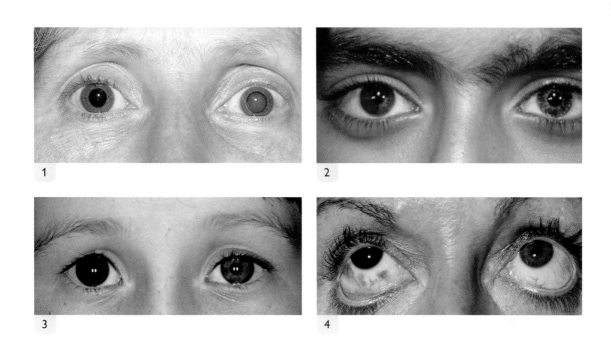

1

2

3

4

Answer on page 65

Q 27 Match (1–3) with the gonioscopy (A–C)

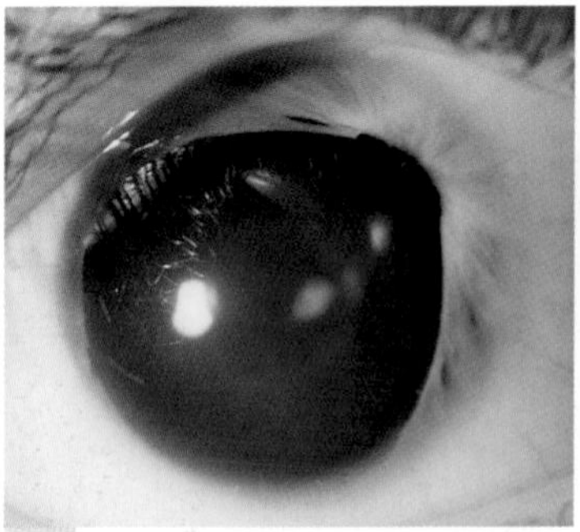

1

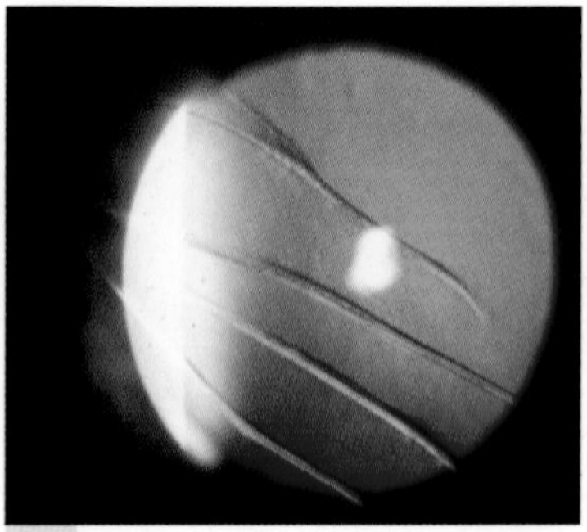

2

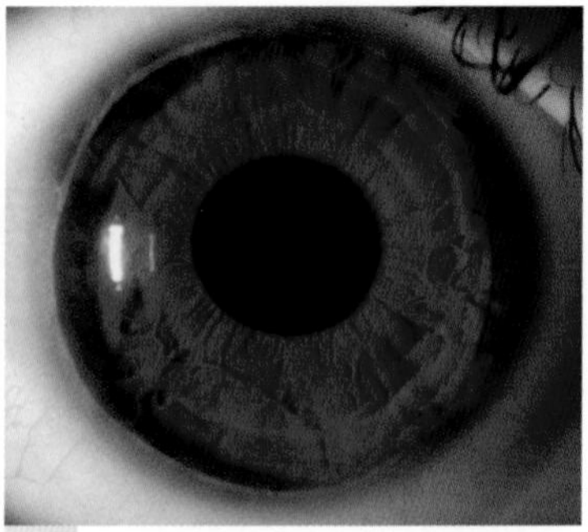

3

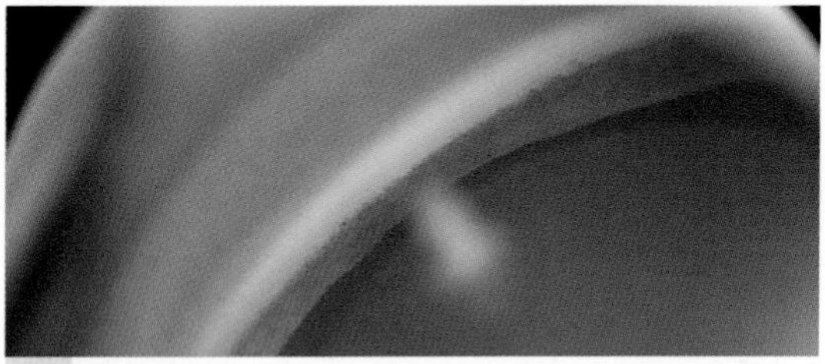

A

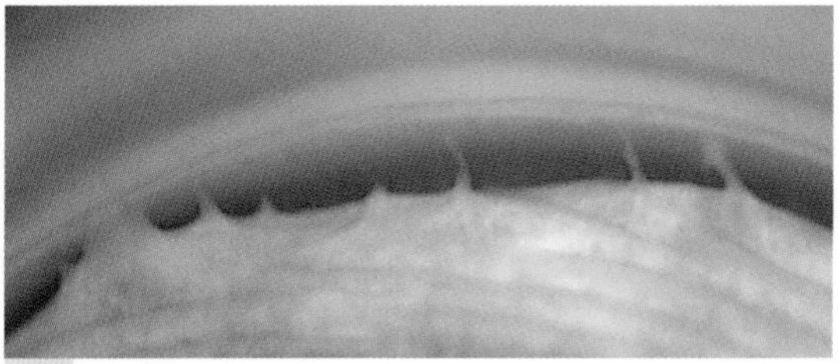

B

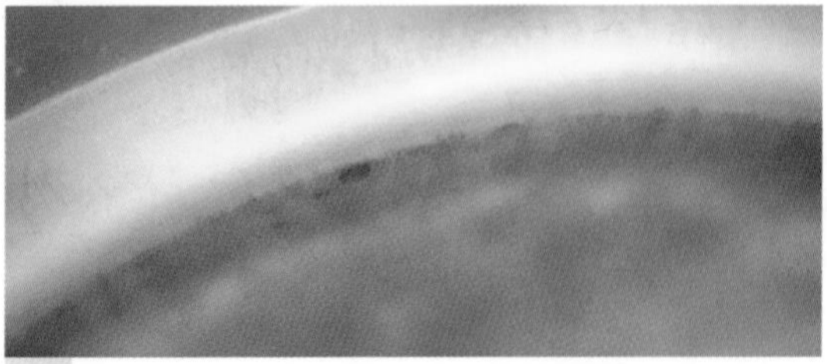

C

Answer on page 66

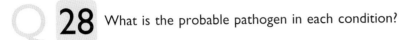

Q 28 What is the probable pathogen in each condition?

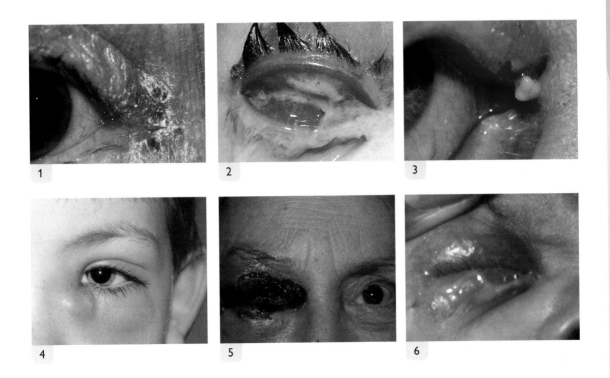

1

2

3

4

5

6

Answer on pages 66–67

Q 29 What is this metabolic disease?

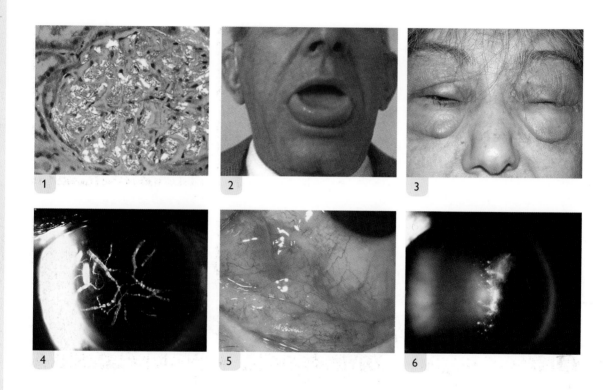

Answer on page 67

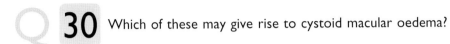
Q 30 Which of these may give rise to cystoid macular oedema?

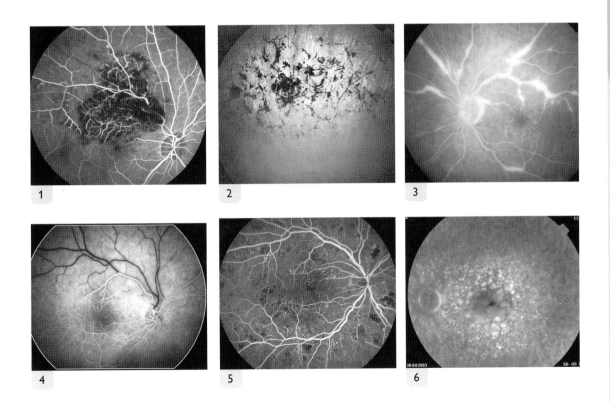

1

2

3

4

5

6

Answer on pages 67–68

Q 31 Which three physicians described these conditions?

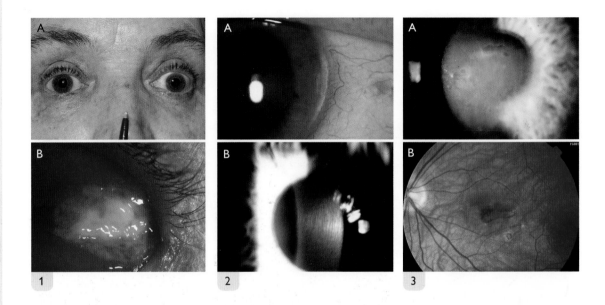

Answer on page 68

Q 32 Which pathogens are responsible for these conditions?

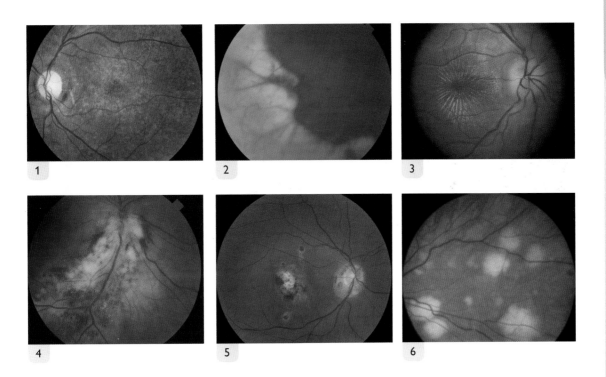

1

2

3

4

5

6

Answer on pages 68–69

Q 33 What are these associations of pigmentary retinopathy?

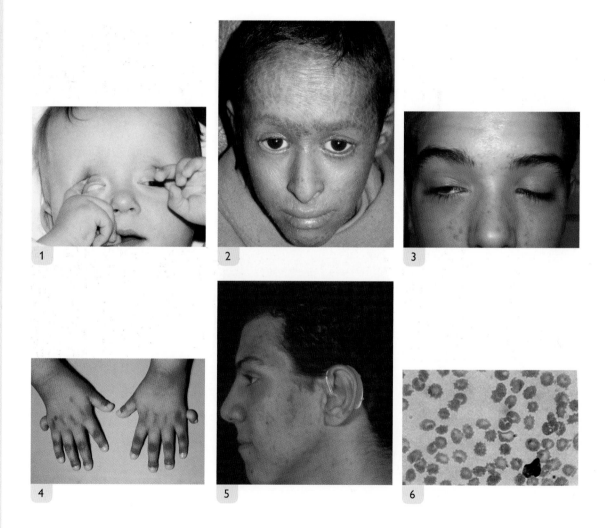

Answer on pages 69–70

Q 34 Match the eyelid tumour (1–3) with the histology (A–C)

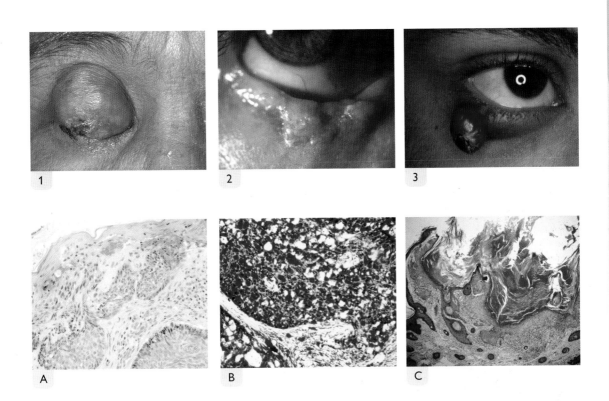

Answer on page 70

35

Q **35** Match (1) with the skin rash (A–D)

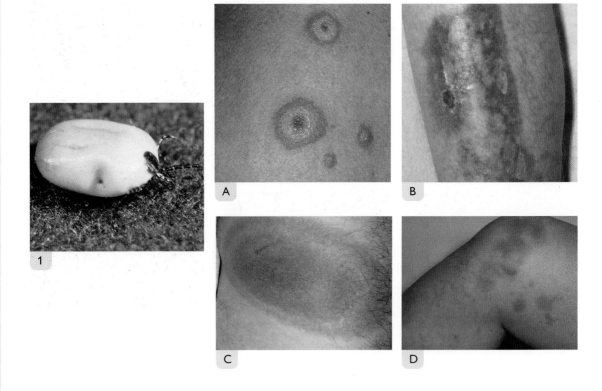

Answer on pages 70–71

Q 36 Match the gonioscopy (1–3) with the pathology (A–C)

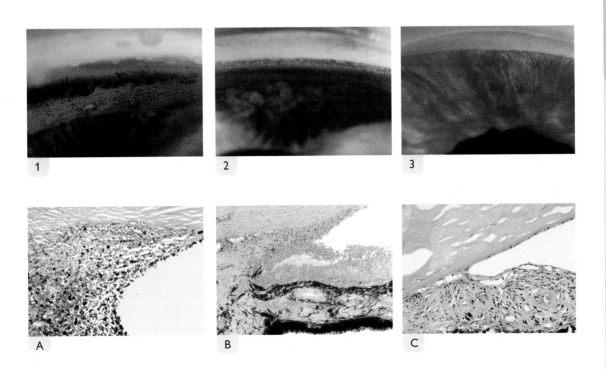

Answer on page 71

Q **37** What do these red reflexes show?

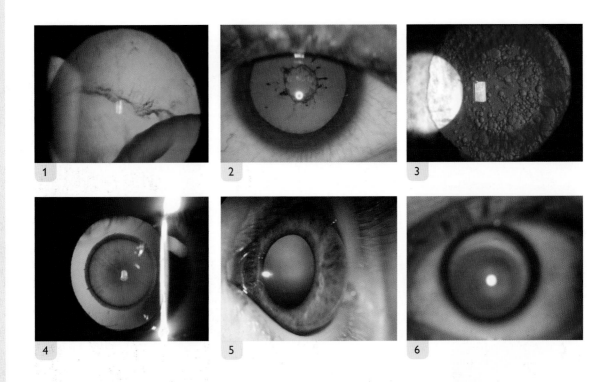

Answer on pages 71–72

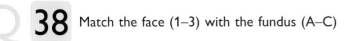

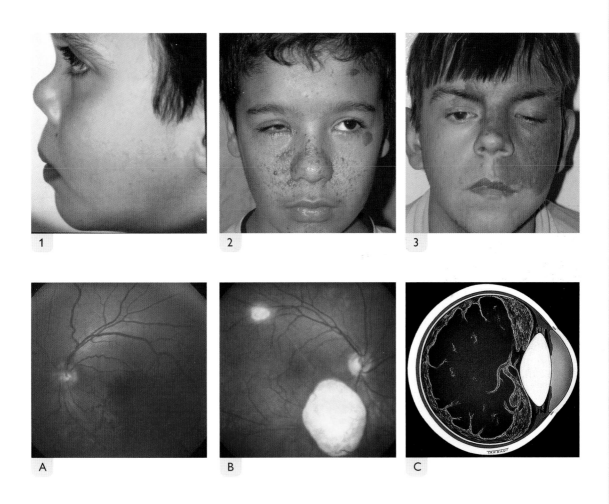

Answer on page 72

Q 39 Which of (A–D) is not associated with 1?

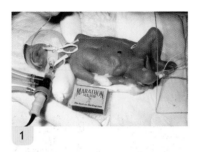

1

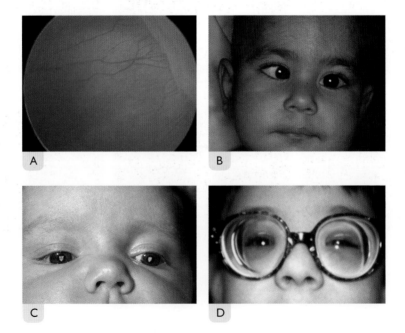

A

B

C

D

Answer on pages 72–73

Q **40** Which is the odd one out?

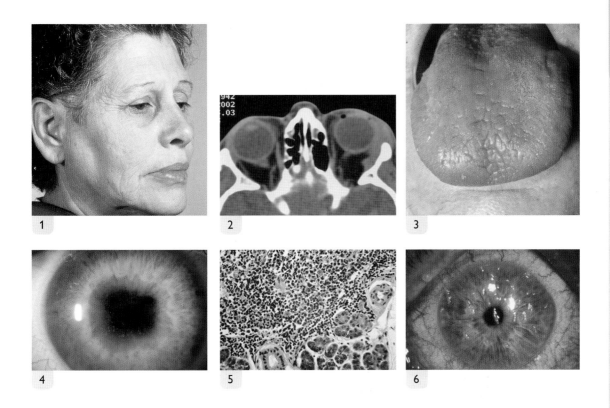

1

2

3

4

5

6

Answer on page 73

Q 41 What multiple pathology is present in these conditions?

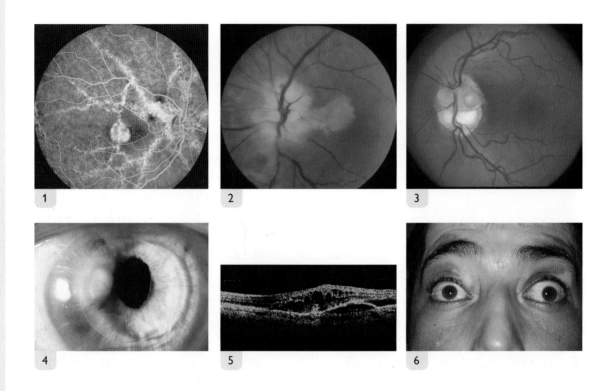

1

2

3

4

5

6

Answer on page 73

Q 42 What treatment has caused these complications?

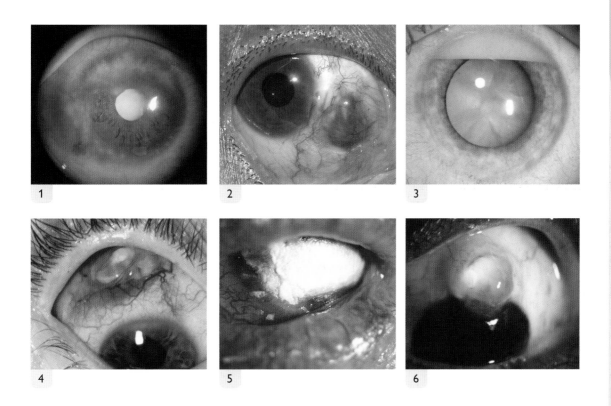

1
2
3
4
5
6

Answer on page 74

Q 43 What do these red-free images show?

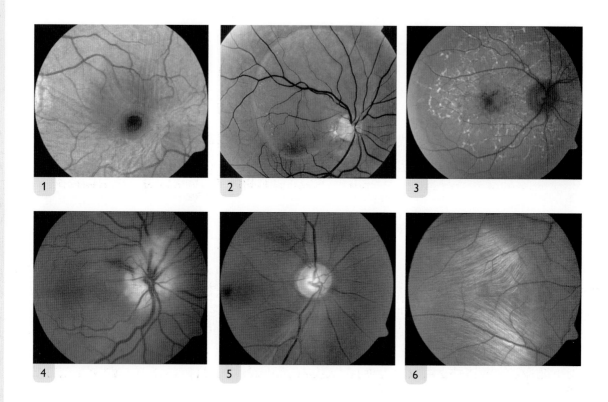

Answer on pages 74–75

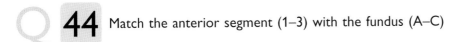
Q 44 Match the anterior segment (1–3) with the fundus (A–C)

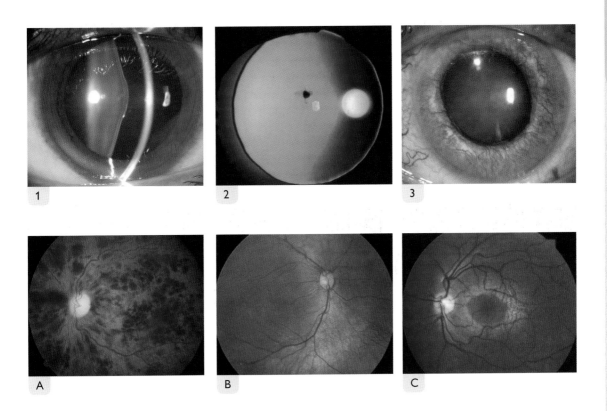

Answer on page 75

SECTION 2

SECTION 3

SECTION 4

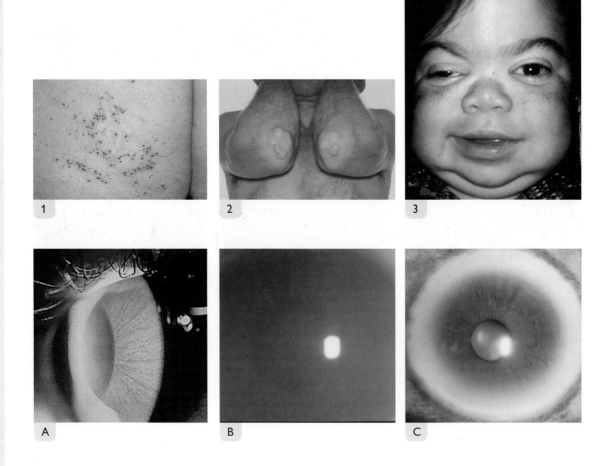

Answer on pages 75–76

Q 46 Who invented these operations?

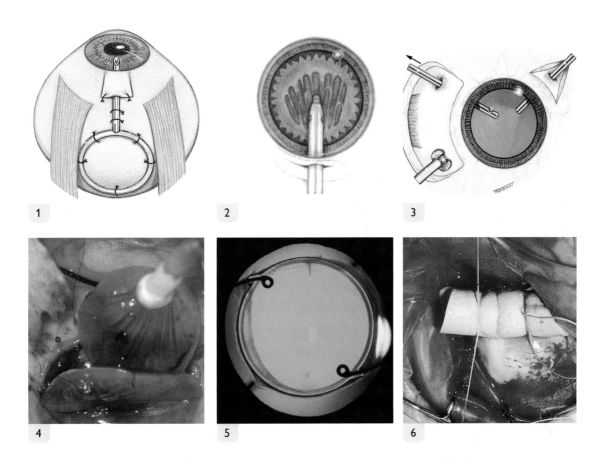

1

2

3

4

5

6

Answer on page 76

Q 47 Match the orbital disorder (1–3) with the CT (A–C)

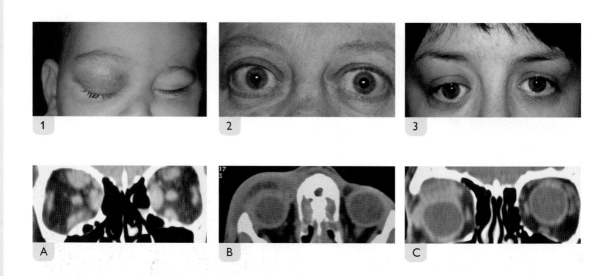

Answer on page 76

Q **48** What are these colour vision tests?

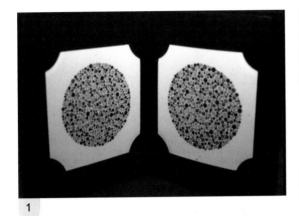

1

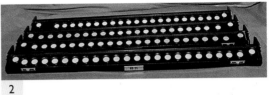

2

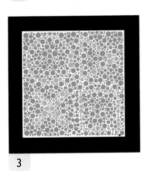

3

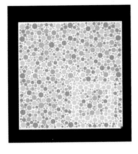

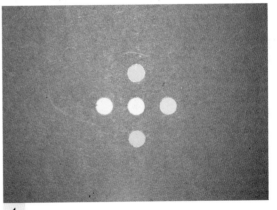

4

Answer on pages 76–77

49 What are these eponymous eyelid procedures?

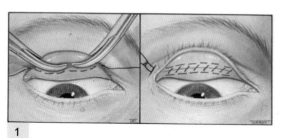

1

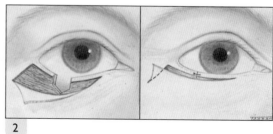

2

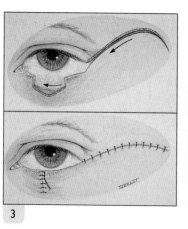

3

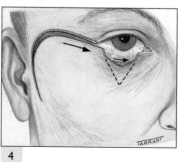

4

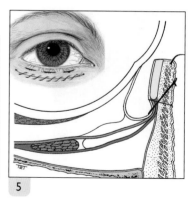

5

Answer on page 77

Q 50 What are these signs?

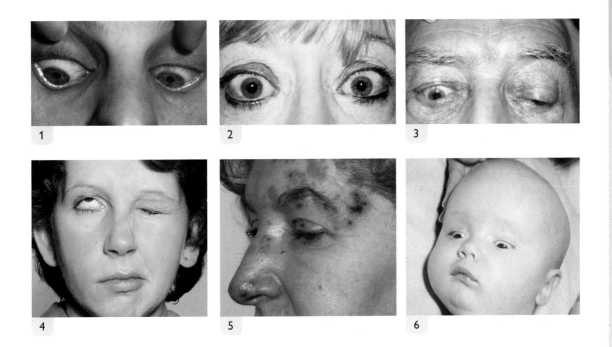

1

2

3

4

5

6

Answer on pages 77–78

1 Answers

1 to 50

Match 1 with one of (A–D)

I and A

Familial adenomatous polyposis (FAP) is an AD condition characterized by polyps throughout the rectum and colon (**1**). If untreated, virtually all patients will develop carcinoma of the colorectal region by the age of 50 years. **Atypical congenital hypertrophy of the RPE** (CHRPE) is present in over 80% of patients with FAP. The lesions are multiple, bilateral, widely separated, frequently spindle-shaped, and with hypopigmentation at one margin (arrow **A**). A positive criterion for FAP is the presence of at least four lesions of whatever size, or at least two lesions – one of which must be large.

Typical grouped CHRPE is characterized by usually unilateral, variably sized, sharply circumscribed, round, oval dark-grey or black lesions, often organized in a pattern simulating animal footprints (bear-track pigmentation – **B**). The lesions are often confined to one sector or quadrant of the fundus with the smaller spots usually located more centrally.

Typical solitary CHRPE is a unilateral, flat, dark-grey or black, well-demarcated, round lesion frequently with a hypopigmented rim within its outer margin (**C**).

Choroidal naevus is an oval or circular, slate-blue or green-grey lesion with detectable but not sharp borders, which may be associated with surface drusen (**D**).

Match the fundus (1–3) with the CT (A–C)

I and B

Optic disc drusen are composed of hyaline-like calcific material within the substance of the optic nerve head. In early childhood drusen may be difficult to detect because they lie deep beneath the surface of the disc. In this setting the appearance may mimic papilloedema. During the early teens drusen usually emerge onto the surface of the disc as waxy pearl-like irregularities (**1**). Imaging may be necessary for the definitive diagnosis of disc drusen, particularly when buried. Ultrasonography is the most readily available and reliable method because of its ability to detect calcific deposits that show high acoustic reflectivity. **CT** shows disc calcification (**B**) but is less sensitive than ultrasonography and may miss small lesions.

2 and A

Choroidal osseous choristoma (osteoma) is a very rare, benign, slow-growing, tumour which is more common in females. Both eyes are affected in about 25% of cases but not usually simultaneously. Presentation is in the second to third decades with gradual visual impairment if the macula is involved by the tumour itself or by secondary choroidal neovascularization. The tumour is orange-yellow, with well-defined, scalloped borders and is located near the disc or at the posterior pole (**2**). **CT** demonstrates bone-like features (**A**).

3 and C

Retinoblastoma is the most common primary, intraocular malignancy of childhood. Growth pattern may be into the vitreous (endophytic – **3**), or into the sub-retinal space (exophytic), causing retinal detachment. Ultrasonography is used mainly to assess tumour size. It also detects calcification within the tumour and is helpful in the diagnosis of simulating lesions such as Coats' disease. **CT** also detects calcification (**C**) but entails a significant dose of radiation and is performed only if ultrasonography has not detected calcification.

QUESTION 3

What do these fluorescein angiograms show?

1. Retinal pigment epithelial detachment is thought to be caused by reduction of hydraulic conductivity of the thickened Bruch membrane, thus impeding movement of fluid from the RPE towards the choroid. FA shows a well demarcated oval area of hyperfluorescence which increases in density but not in size throughout the angiogram due to pooling of dye under the detachment.

2. Cystoid macular oedema is the result of accumulation of fluid in the outer plexiform and inner nuclear layers of the retina with the formation of fluid-filled cyst-like changes. The arteriovenous phase shows small hyperfluorescent spots due to early leakage; the late venous phase shows increasing hyperfluorescence and coalescence of the focal leaks; the recirculation phase shows a 'flower-petal' pattern of hyperfluorescence caused by accumulation of dye within microcystic spaces in the outer plexiform layer of the retina, with its radial arrangement of fibres about the centre of the foveola (Henle layer).

3. Central serous retinopathy is a disorder of the outer blood–retinal barrier, characterized by a localized detachment of the sensory retina at the macula secondary to focal RPE defects, usually affecting one eye. Early FA typically shows a small hyperfluorescent spot due to leakage of dye through the RPE. During the late venous phase, the dye passes into the subretinal space and ascends vertically (like a smoke-stack) up to the upper border of the detachment, and then spreads laterally until the entire area is filled.

4. Choroidal neovascularization (CNV) is an important cause of visual morbidity in elderly patients with wet macular degeneration. The CNV originates in the choriocapillaris and then grows into the sub-RPE space through defects in Bruch membrane. Classic CNV is a well-defined membrane which fills with dye in a 'lacy' pattern during the very early phase of dye transit, fluoresces brightly during peak dye transit, and then leaks into the sub-retinal space and around the CNV within 1–2 min. Staining of the fibrous tissue within the CNV results in late hyperfluorescence.

QUESTION 4

Herpes simplex or herpes zoster?

1. Herpes simplex rash typically affects children with primary infection (no previous exposure). It is occasionally bilateral but asymmetrical. The vesicles break down within 48 hours and resolve without residua. Secondary conjunctivitis may occur but corneal involvement is rare.

2. Herpes zoster keratitis is characterized by fine dendritic lesions with tapered endings that do not contain terminal bulbs; they stain with fluorescein and Rose Bengal.

3. Herpes zoster ophthalmicus (HZO) typically affects elderly individuals but may occasionally affect children, particularly with compromised immunity. The lesions are unilateral and confined to the cutaneous distribution of the first division of the trigeminal nerve.

4. Herpes simplex dendritic ulceration is characterized by a linear-branching ulcer, most frequently located centrally. The ends of the ulcer have characteristic terminal buds and the bed of the ulcer stains well with fluorescein whilst the virus-laden cells at the margin of the ulcer stain with Rose Bengal. Occasionally more than one lesion may be present.

5. Herpes zoster nummular keratitis usually develops about 10 days after the onset of the rash. It is characterized by fine granular subepithelial deposits surrounded by a halo of stromal haze. The lesions fade in response to topical steroids but recur if treatment is discontinued prematurely.

6. Herpes simplex disciform keratitis is characterized by a central zone of stromal oedema often with overlying epithelial oedema with underlying keratic precipitates. Folds in Descemet membrane may be seen in severe cases. A surrounding (Wessely) immune ring of stromal haze is occasionally present and signifies deposition of viral antigen and host antibody complexes.

QUESTION 5

Two systemic diseases are shown: match each ocular sign (1 and 2) with the systemic feature (A–D)

Lepromatous leprosy may result in chronic low-grade anterior uveitis due to direct invasion of the iris by bacilli. A pathognomonic sign is the presence of iris pearls formed from dead bacteria (**1**) that slowly enlarge and coalesce, become pedunculated and then drop into the anterior chamber. Eventually, the pupil becomes miosed and the iris atrophic as a result of damage to the sympathetic innervation to the dilator pupillae. Systemic manifestations include a leonine facies characterized by cutaneous thickening and ridging, nasal widening and thickening of ear lobes, and saddle-shaped nasal deformity (**A**). Motor neuropathy is exemplified by the 'claw hand' deformity due to ulnar nerve palsy (**C**).

Onchocerciasis is caused by the filarial parasite *Onchocerca volvulus* which is transmitted by the bite of a blackfly (Simulium) resulting in the migration of millions of tiny worms (microfilariae) throughout the body. Chorioretinitis is usually bilateral and predominantly involves the posterior fundus. The severity varies from atrophy and clumping of the RPE, which may resemble choroidal 'sclerosis', to widespread chorioretinal atrophy (**2**). Systemic manifestations include subcutaneous nodules (onchocercomas) consisting of encapsulated worms that develop over bony prominences (**B**) and focal areas of cutaneous hypo- and hyperpigmentation on the shins ('leopard' skin – **D**).

What inflammatory conditions do these angiograms show?

1. Harada disease. Vogt–Koyanagi–Harada syndrome is an idiopathic, multisystem, autoimmune disease against melanocytes that results in inflammation of melanocyte-containing tissues such as the uvea, ears, skin, and meninges. It can be subdivided into Vogt–Koyanagi disease, which predominantly affects the skin and is associated with granulomatous anterior uveitis, and Harada disease, which is characterized by neurological features and bilateral exudative retinal detachments. **FA** initially shows multifocal hyperfluorescent dots at the level of the RPE (**A**) followed by accumulation of dye in the subretinal space (**B**).

2. Multiple evanescent white dot syndrome is an uncommon, idiopathic, usually unilateral, self-limiting disease which typically affects individuals between the ages of 20–40 years, particularly females. **FA** shows subtle punctate hyperfluorescence some of which may form a cluster or 'wreath-shaped' pattern (**A**). **ICG** shows more numerous hypofluorescent spots (**B**) than are apparent clinically or on FA.

3. Acute posterior multifocal placoid pigment epitheliopathy is an uncommon, idiopathic, usually bilateral condition, which typically affects individuals in the third to sixth decades. It affects both sexes equally and is associated with HLA-B7 and HLA-DR2. **FA** of active lesions shows early dense hypofluorescence associated with non-perfusion of the choriocapillaris (**A**) and late hyperfluorescence due to staining (**B**).

Match the uveitis (1–3) with the pathogen (A–C)

1 and A

Toxocariasis is caused by infestation with a common intestinal ascarid (roundworm) of dogs called *Toxocara canis* (**A**). About 80% of puppies between the ages of 2 and 6 months are infested. Human infestation is by accidental ingestion of soil or food contaminated with ova shed in dog faeces. Ocular involvement is invariably unilateral and occurs in patients without systemic manifestations. The three main manifestations are: chronic endophthalmitis that may cause leukocoria, a peripheral granuloma that may cause 'dragging' of the disc and macula, or a white granuloma at the posterior fundus (**1**).

2 and C

Toxoplasmosis is caused by *Toxoplasma gondii*, an obligate intracellular protozoan. It is the most frequent cause of infectious retinitis in immunocompetent individuals. Although some cases may occur as a result of reactivation of prenatal infestation the vast majority are acquired postnatally. Fundoscopy typically shows a solitary inflammatory focus near an old pigmented scar ('satellite lesion' – **2**). Recurrent episodes of inflammation are common and occur when the cysts rupture and release hundreds of tachyzoites into normal retinal cells (**C**).

3 and B

Candidiasis is caused by metastatic spread from a septic focus associated with catheters, intravenous drug abuse, parenteral nutrition, and chronic lung disease such as cystic fibrosis. Neutropenia following immunosuppression and AIDS are also major risk factors. Ocular infection is characterized by creamy white chorioretinal lesions with overlying vitritis, often associated with floating 'cotton-ball' vitreous opacities (**3**). Vitreous biopsy and smears showing pseudo-hyphae ('germ tubes' – **B**) is required to confirm the diagnosis.

QUESTION 8

Match the keratic precipitates (1–3) with (A–C)

1 and C

Acute anterior uveitis has a sudden onset and a duration of 3 months or less. Endothelial dusting by myriad of cells is present early and gives rise to a 'dirty' appearance (**1**). The injection is circumcorneal (ciliary) with a violaceous hue, and the pupil is miosed (**C**) due to sphincter spasm that may predispose to the formation of posterior synechiae. Important causes of acute anterior uveitis include: HLA-B27 associated spondyloarthropathies, inflammatory bowel disease, acute-onset sarcoidosis, Behçet disease, syphilis, and relapsing polychondritis.

2 and B

Fuchs uveitis syndrome is a chronic anterior uveitis of insidious onset. The keratic precipitates are characteristically small, round or stellate, grey-white in colour and scattered throughout the corneal endothelium (**2**). The iris stroma becomes progressively atrophic and small nodules may be seen at the papillary border. Advanced stromal atrophy makes the affected iris appear dull with loss of detail giving rise to a washed-out appearance, particularly in the pupillary zone (**B**).

3 and A

Granulomatous anterior uveitis is characterized by large keratic precipitates that have a greasy ('mutton-fat') appearance. They are often more numerous inferiorly and may form in a triangular pattern with the apex pointing up (**3**). Iris nodules are of three types: Koeppe nodules are small and situated at the pupillary border; Busacca nodules are stromal; and large pink nodules (**A**) that are characteristic of sarcoid uveitis. Important causes of granulomatous uveitis include: sarcoidosis, Vogt–Harada–Koyanagi syndrome, sympathetic ophthalmitis, syphilis, and toxoplasmosis.

QUESTION 9

Match the hands (1–3) with the eye (A–C)

1 and B

Psoriatic arthritis affects a minority of patients with psoriasis who also show nail dystrophy characterized by pitting, transverse depression, and onycholysis. Arthritis involving the hands is often asymmetrical and involves the distal interphalangeal joints (**1**). **Acute anterior uveitis**, which may give rise to posterior synechiae (**B**), is uncommon except in patients with co-existing ankylosing spondylitis.

2 and A

Marfan syndrome is a widespread AD disorder of connective tissue associated with mutation of the fibrillin gene. Patients are tall and thin, with disproportionately long limbs compared with the trunk (arm span > height), and have long spider-like fingers and toes (arachnodactyly – **2**). **Ectopia lentis**, which is bilateral and symmetrical, is present in 80% of cases. Subluxation is most frequently superotemporal (**A**), but may be in any meridian. Because the zonule is frequently intact, accommodation is retained, although rarely the lens may become totally dislocated.

3 and C

Rheumatoid arthritis (RA) is an autoimmune systemic disease characterized by inflammatory polyarthropathy association with a spectrum of extra-articular manifestations. Symmetrical arthritis of the small joints of the hands typically involves the proximal interphalangeal and spares the distal interphalangeal joints (**3**). RA is by far the most common systemic association of **scleritis**. Patients with non-necrotizing disease (**C**) usually have mild joint involvement, whereas necrotizing scleritis tends to affect patients with severe long-standing RA.

QUESTION 10

Match the face (1–3) with the iris (A–C)

1 and C

Blunt ocular trauma has caused a left blow-out fracture with entrapment of the inferior rectus muscle that has prevented elevation (**1**). **Dialysis of the iris** can also be caused by blunt ocular trauma (**C**).

2 and A

Neurofibromatosis-1 (NF-1) is a disorder that primarily affects cell growth of neural tissues. Inheritance is AD with irregular penetrance and variable expressivity. Discrete small cutaneous neurofibromas may involve the face, and plexiform neurofibromas involving the eyelids give rise to the characteristic S-shaped deformities (**2**). **Lisch nodules** are small, bilateral, iris naevi (**A**) found after the age of 16 years in virtually all patients with NF-1.

3 and B

Down syndrome (trisomy 21) is characterized by upward-slanting palpebral fissures, epicanthic folds, and midfacial flattening (**3**). Other features include mental handicap, brachycephalic skull with flattening of the occiput, broad short hands, and a protruding tongue. **Brushfield spots** are pale lesions in the peripheral stroma (**B**) that may be found in some normal individuals as well as in the majority of patients with Down syndrome. Cataract of varying morphology occurs in about 75% of patients. The opacities are usually symmetrical and often develop in late childhood.

QUESTION 11

What are the wild animal connotations?

1. Panda eyes are bilateral traumatic periorbital haematomas that may be associated with a basal skull fracture.

2. Crocodile shagreen is characterized by asymptomatic, greyish-white, polygonal stromal opacities separated by relatively clear spaces. The opacities most frequently involve the anterior two-thirds of the stroma (anterior crocodile shagreen), although on occasion they may be found more posteriorly (posterior crocodile shagreen).

3. Elephantiasis nervosa occurs in patients with neurofibromatosis-1 when infiltration by a diffuse plexiform neurofibroma causes overgrowth of soft tissue and thick redundant skin, resulting in severe disfigurement.

4. Polar-bear track is a rare innocuous condition characterized by multiple, grouped, round or oval areas of atrophic RPE.

5. Serpiginous choroidopathy is an uncommon, chronic, recurrent, inflammatory disease affecting individuals in the fourth to sixth decades of life. It affects men more than women and is associated with HLA-B7. Active lesions are grey-white to yellow in appearance and are located at the level of the RPE or inner choroid. Inactive lesions are characterized by scalloped, atrophic, 'punched-out' areas of choroidal and RPE atrophy.

6. Leopard-spots consist of scattered areas of sub-retinal pigmentary mottling that may develop following resolution of an exudative retinal detachment or uveal effusion syndrome. 'Shifting fluid' is the hallmark of exudative retinal detachment in which very mobile subretinal fluid responds to the force of gravity and detaches the area of retina under which it accumulates.

QUESTION 12

What are the animal connotations?

1. Rodent ulcer (noduloulcerative) basal cell carcinoma is characterized by central ulceration, pearly raised rolled edges with dilated and irregular blood vessels over its lateral margins. It gradually enlarges, and with time, may erode a large portion of the eyelid and underlying tissues.

2. Butterfly dystrophy is one of the pattern dystrophies characterized by bilateral, symmetrical, yellow, orange or grey deposits at the macula that have a variety of morphologies. In butterfly dystrophy the lesions are arranged in a triradiate manner. Inheritance is AD, the ERG is normal and the long-term prognosis usually good.

3. Bull's eye maculopathy is characterized by a central foveolar island of pigment surrounded by a depigmented zone of RPE atrophy, which is itself encircled by a hyperpigmented ring. FA shows hyperfluorescence due to a window defect that corresponds to the RPE atrophy.

4. Cattle-trucking describes sludging and segmentation of the blood column in association with acute retinal arterial occlusion.

5. Snailtrack is a peripheral retinal degeneration characterized by sharply demarcated bands of tightly packed 'snowflakes' which give the peripheral retina a white frost-like appearance. Round holes may be present within the lesions. The bands are usually longer than islands of lattice degeneration and may be associated with overlying vitreous liquefaction.

6. Salmon patches occur in non-proliferative sickle cell retinopathy. They consist of pink, preretinal or superficial intraretinal haemorrhages at the equator. They lie adjacent to arterioles and usually resolve without sequelae.

QUESTION 13

Which of these are not associated with recurrent corneal erosions?

5 Macular dystrophy

1. A corneal abrasion is a breach of the epithelium which stains with fluorescein. Recurrent corneal epithelial **erosions** is the tendency for minor trauma to cause ocular pain or an epithelial defect following healing of a corneal abrasion. Opening the eye after sleep can cause shearing forces sufficient to cause movement of the epithelial sheet or tearing of the epithelium.

2. Reis–Bückler dystrophy presents in first or second decade with painful recurrent corneal

erosions. It is an AD condition characterized by grey-white, fine, round and polygonal opacities in Bowman layer, most dense centrally.

3. Epithelial basement membrane dystrophy (Cogan microcystic, map-dot-fingerprint dystrophy) is the most common dystrophy seen in clinical practice. The vast majority of cases are sporadic. About 10% of patients develop recurrent corneal erosions in the third decade. Simultaneous bilateral recurrent **erosions** suggest epithelial basement membrane dystrophy. The following lesions may be seen in isolation or combination: dot-like opacities, epithelial microcysts, subepithelial map-like patterns surrounded by a faint haze, and whorled fingerprint-like lines.

4. Granular dystrophy is occasionally associated with recurrent corneal **erosions**. It is an AD condition characterized by small, white, sharply demarcated deposits resembling crumbs, rings or snowflakes in the central anterior stroma.

5. Macular dystrophy is the least common stromal dystrophy in which a systemic inborn error of keratan sulphate metabolism has only corneal manifestations. Onset is towards the end of the first decade with gradual visual deterioration but corneal erosions do not occur. It is an AR condition characterized by a central anterior stromal haze and dense, focal greyish-white, poorly delineated spots in the anterior stroma centrally and posterior stroma in the periphery.

6. Lattice dystrophy presents at the end of the first decade with recurrent **erosions**. It is an AD condition characterized by stromal lattice lines and haze. Recurrent erosions may precede the typical stromal changes so that the condition may be missed.

QUESTION 14

What is the probable associated refraction?

1. Choroidal folds are parallel grooves or striae at the posterior pole. Possible mechanisms include choroidal congestion, scleral folding, and contraction of Bruch membrane. Idiopathic folds may affect both eyes of healthy **hypermetropic** patients with normal or near-normal visual acuity. Other causes of choroidal folds include orbital disease, choroidal tumours, posterior scleritis, scleral buckling, and chronic papilloedema.

2. Refractive accommodative esotropia is a physiological response to excessive **hypermetropia**, usually between +2.00 and +7.00 D. The considerable degree of accommodation required to focus is accompanied by a proportionate amount of convergence, which is beyond the patient's fusional divergence amplitude. It cannot therefore be controlled, and a manifest convergent squint results. Fully accommodative esotropia is eliminated by optical correction of hypermetropia. Constant accommodative esotropia is reduced, but not eliminated by full correction of hypermetropia.

3. Tilted disc and chorioretinal atrophy typically develop in **highly myopic** eyes in which the axial length of the globe is over 26 mm.

4. Cornea plana is a rare, hereditary, bilateral condition in which the corneal curvature is significantly reduced with associated reduction of corneal refractive power. It is characterized by severe **hypermetropia**, shallow anterior chamber, and predisposition to angle closure. Ocular associations include microcornea, sclerocornea, microphthalmos, and Peters anomaly.

5. Keratoconus is a progressive disorder in which the cornea assumes a conical shape secondary to stromal thinning and protrusion. Presentation is typically during puberty with unilateral impairment of vision due to progressive **myopia and astigmatism**. The latter subsequently becomes irregular.

6. Nuclear cataract starts as an exaggeration of the normal ageing changes involving the lens nucleus. It is often associated with **myopia** due to an increase in the refractive index of the lens nucleus and also with increased spherical aberration. Some elderly patients may consequently be able to read again without spectacles ('second sight of the aged'). Nuclear sclerosis is characterized in its early stages by a yellowish hue due to the deposition of urochrome pigment; when advanced the nucleus appears brown (brunescent cataract).

QUESTION 15

What is this condition?

Floppy eyelid syndrome is an uncommon, unilateral or bilateral condition, which typically affects middle-aged, obese men who sleep face down with their lids everted by the pillow. Nocturnal exposure and poor contact of the lax lid with the globe in combination with tear film abnormalities results in chronic papillary conjunctivitis affecting the superior tarsal conjunctiva as well as keratitis of varying severity. Affected patients typically have redundant upper lid skin, and loose and rubbery tarsal plates that evert with ease.

QUESTION 16

Match the face (1–3) with the cataract (A–C)

I and B

Myotonic dystrophy (dystrophia myotonica, Steinert disease) is an AD disease characterized by delayed muscular relaxation after cessation of voluntary effort (myotonia). Facial features include ptosis, a mournful expression caused by bilateral facial wasting with hollow cheeks, and frontal baldness in males (**1**). About 90% of patients develop visually insignificant, fine cortical iridescent opacities in the third decade, which evolve into visually disabling **stellate posterior subcapsular cataract** (**B**) by the fifth decade. Occasionally cataract may antedate myotonia.

2 and A

Cushing syndrome is due to prolonged elevation of free plasma glucocorticoid levels. The most common cause is iatrogenic due to systemic administration of steroids. The face becomes swollen (moon face) and the complexion plethoric (**2**). Steroids, both systemic and topical, are cataractogenic. The lens opacities are initially **posterior subcapsular** (**A**). The relationship between weekly systemic dose, duration of administration, total dose, and cataract formation is unclear although it is thought that patients on less than 10 mg prednisolone (or equivalent), or treated for less than 4 years may be immune. It is believed that children may be more susceptible than adults.

3 and C

Atopic eczema (dermatitis) is an idiopathic, often familial, condition, which may be associated with asthma and hay fever. Facial eczema is characterized by itchy, dry, erythematous papules, often associated with madarosis and staphylococcal blepharitis

(**3**). About 10% of patients with severe atopic dermatitis develop **shield-like dense anterior subcapsular plaques** which wrinkle the anterior capsule (**C**). They are often bilateral and may mature quickly. Other associations of atopic eczema are chronic keratoconjunctivitis, keratoconus, and rarely, retinal detachment.

QUESTION 17

Match the drug side-effect (1–3) with the indication for its use (A–C)

I and B

Chloroquine is used in the treatment of connective tissue diseases such as systemic lupus erythematosus, characterized by a facial rash with a butterfly distribution (**B**). **Vortex keratopathy** (**1**) may develop in some patients. It is innocuous, not dose-related, and usually reversible on cessation of therapy.

2 and C

Strong miotics are occasionally used short-term in the treatment of accommodative esotropia due to a high AC/A ratio (**C**). Their use may cause the formation of **iris cysts** at the papillary border (**2**) unless 2.5% phenylephrine is administered simultaneously.

3 and A

Tamoxifen is a specific anti-oestrogen used in the treatment of selected patients with breast carcinoma (**A**). The normal daily dose is 20–40 mg. Retinotoxicity and visual impairment may develop in some patients on higher doses, and rarely, on normal doses. Retinopathy is characterized by bilateral, fine, superficial, yellow, **crystalline deposits** at the posterior pole (**3**).

QUESTION 18

Match the fundus dystrophy (1–3) with the findings in carriers (A–C)

I and B

Albinism is a genetically determined, heterogeneous group of disorders of melanin synthesis in which either the eyes alone (ocular albinism) or the eyes, skin, and hair (oculocutaneous albinism) may be affected. The latter may be either tyrosinase-positive or tyrosinase-negative. The fundus lacks pigment and shows conspicuously large choroidal vessels. There is also foveal hypoplasia and lack of vessels forming the perimacular arcades (**1**). **Female carriers of ocular albinism** are asymptomatic although they may show partial iris translucency, macular stippling, and mid-peripheral scattered areas of depigmentation and granularity (**B**).

2 and A

Choroideremia is a XLR diffuse degeneration of the choroid, RPE, and photoreceptors. Fundoscopy shows atrophy of the choriocapillaris and choroid rendering visible underlying sclera (**2**). In contrast to primary retinal dystrophies, the fovea is spared until late and the optic disc and retinal blood vessels remain relatively normal. **Female carriers** show mild, patchy peripheral RPE atrophy and mottling (**A**).

3 and C

Retinitis pigmentosa (RP) defines a clinically and genetically diverse group of diffuse retinal dystrophies initially predominantly affecting the rod photoreceptor cells with subsequent degeneration of cones. The classic clinical triad of RP is: arteriolar attenuation, retinal bone-spicule pigmentation, and waxy disc pallor (**3**). XL is the least common but most severe form which may result in complete blindness by the third or fourth decades. **Female carriers** may have normal fundi or exhibit a golden-metallic reflex at the macula (**C**).

the nuclear remnant to the edge of the cell. The bodies are small and eosinophilic near the surface and large and basophilic deeper down (**A**). Lesions on the lid margin may shed virus into the tear film and give rise to secondary, ipsilateral, chronic, follicular conjunctivitis.

QUESTION 19

Match the eyelid lesion (1–3) with the histology (A–C)

1 and B

Squamous cell papilloma (fibroepithelial polyp) is a very common condition. The lesion may be pedunculated (**1**), sessile, or hyperkeratotic. **Histology** common to all three types are finger-like projections of fibrovascular connective tissue covered by irregular acanthotic and hyperkeratotic squamous epithelium (**B**).

2 and C

Epidermoid (keratinous) cyst results from implantation of surface epidermis during trauma or surgery, and appears as a firm, round, mobile lesion which may be superficial or subcutaneous (**2**). **Histology** shows a keratin-filled cavity within the dermis lined by stratified squamous epithelium (**C**). The term 'sebaceous' cyst is often incorrectly used to describe this lesion.

3 and A

Molluscum contagiosum is a skin infection caused by a human specific double stranded DNA poxvirus which typically affects otherwise healthy children. The lesion consists of a pale, waxy umbilicated nodule. Multiple, and occasionally confluent, lesions (**3**) may develop in immunocompromised patients. **Histology** shows lobules of hyperplastic epidermis with intracytoplasmic inclusion bodies that displace

QUESTION 20

Match the retinal detachment (1–3) with the ultrasonogram (A–C)

1 and B

Exudative retinal detachment due to a choroidal melanoma is smooth, bullous and has deep subretinal fluid (**1**). **Ultrasonography** shows a mushroom-shaped tumour with retinal separation inferiorly. The lesion contains an area of acoustic hollowness and choroidal excavation (a dark appearance in the normally highly reflective choroid) (**B**). Exudative RD tends to be very mobile and exhibits the phenomenon of 'shifting fluid'. Apart from tumours causes include Harada disease, toxaemia of pregnancy, uveal effusion syndrome, and bullous central serous retinopathy.

2 and C

Rhegmatogenous retinal detachment is convex and shows retinal wrinkling due to early proliferative vitreoretinopathy (**2**). **Ultrasonography** shows a funnel-shaped detachment attached to the optic nerve head with some wrinkling of the retinal surface (**C**).

3 and A

Tractional retinal detachment has a concave shape, is associated with severe fibrovascular proliferation, and is relatively immobile (**3**). **Ultrasonog-**

raphy shows a tabletop detachment attached to the optic nerve head by a stalk; intragel haemorrhage is also present (**A**). Important causes are proliferative diabetic retinopathy and penetrating trauma.

QUESTION 21

Match (1–3) with the gonioscopy (A–C)

I and C

Progressive iris atrophy typically affects one eye of a middle-aged female. It is characterized by corectopia, iris stromal atrophy, and full-thickness iris defects (**1**). **Gonioscopy** shows broad-based peripheral anterior synechiae extending anterior to Schwalbe line (**C**). Progressive iris atrophy forms part of the iridocorneal endothelial syndrome (ICE); the other two are iris naevus (Cogan–Reese) syndrome and Chandler syndrome.

2 and B

Post-congestive angle closure manifests iris atrophy, a dilated pupil, posterior synechiae, and small, anterior lens opacities (glaukomflecken) (**2**). **Gonioscopy** shows complete angle closure (**B**). The other stages of angle-closure are intermittent, acute congestive, and chronic.

3 and A

Secondary inflammatory angle-closure without pupillary block. Posterior synechiae are present despite treatment with mydriatics (**3**). **Gonioscopy** shows angle closure by several broad-based peripheral anterior synechiae (**A**). Secondary inflammatory glaucoma is a common cause of permanent visual loss in children with chronic anterior uveitis.

QUESTION 22

What are these complications of vitreoretinal surgery?

1. Infection of an encircling element may rarely occur when it becomes exposed several months or weeks postoperatively. This is usually the result of inadequate coverage with Tenon capsule and conjunctiva during surgery.

2. Subretinal injection of gas is an extremely rare complication that may occur when gas is used to tamponade a large retinal break.

3. Erosion of an explant through the eyelid is an extremely rare complication caused by inadequate suturing of the sponge to the sclera.

4. Haemorrhage is usually caused by damage to a large choroidal vessel during drainage of subretinal fluid (SRF). Small bleeds may be innocuous because the blood escapes with the SRF. Large bleeds may give rise to postoperative maculopathy as a result of gravitation of blood in the subretinal space to the fovea, as well as vitreous haemorrhage and haemorrhagic choroidal detachment.

5. Retinal incarceration into the sclerotomy is a serious complication usually due to excessively elevated intraocular pressure at the time of drainage using the 'cut-down' technique. Management is very difficult and may require retinotomy.

6. Failure to close a large retinal tear in an eye with proliferative vitreoretinopathy requires re-operation involving vitrectomy.

QUESTION 23

What have these conditions in common?

Optic disc drusen

1. Disc drusen in an eye with **macular drusen**; the two are not related.

2. Drusen in an eye with macular scarring associated with **choroidal neovascularization**; this is a rare but well established association.

3. Disc drusen in an eye with **angioid streaks**; a well known association.

4. Drusen in an eye with inferior disc traction in an eye with a combined **hamartoma** of the retina and RPE; an occasional association.

5. Ultrasonogram of disc drusen which shows high acoustic reflectivity and orbital shadowing.

6. Disc drusen in an eye with **pigmentary retinopathy**; a well-established association.

Other ocular complications of disc drusen include: disc neovascularization, central retinal arterial and venous occlusion, and retinal nerve fibre visual field defects. The only systemic association is Alagille syndrome.

QUESTION 24

Match the conjunctivitis (1–3) with the keratopathy (A–C)

1 and B

Vernal keratoconjunctivitis (VKC) is a bilateral, recurrent, disorder that typically starts in the first decade and usually remits by the late teens. Many patients have associated atopic disease. Superior tarsal papillary conjunctivitis is universal. In severe cases the papillae become large and resemble cobblestone (**1**). Corneal shield ulcers and plaques are uncommon (**B**). They may result in poor wetting and delayed corneal re-epithelialization. Patients with VKC have an increased incidence of keratoconus, frequently complicated by hydrops, and a strong tendency for vascularization.

2 and A

Trachoma is chronic conjunctival inflammation caused by infection with serotypes A, B, Ba, and C of *C. trachomatis*. It is the most common cause of preventable blindness in the world. Chronic disease is characterized by linear or stellate conjunctival scars involving the superior tarsus (**2**) and superior pannus formation (**A**).

3 and C

Adenoviral keratoconjunctivitis is the most common external ocular viral infection that may be sporadic or occur in epidemics. It is characterized by acute follicular conjunctivitis, most severe in the inferior fornix (**3**) and tender pre-auricular lymphadenopathy. Keratitis can be divided into three stages: *Stage 1* is characterized by a punctate epithelial keratitis that resolves within 2 weeks; *Stage 2* manifests focal, white, subepithelial opacities that develop beneath the fading epithelial lesions (**C**); *Stage 3* shows anterior stromal infiltrates that gradually fade over months or years.

Match the blepharitis (1–3) with the dermatitis (A–C)

1 and A

Staphylococcal blepharitis is characterized by hard scales and crusting mainly located around the bases of the lashes. Scarring and notching (tylosis) of the lid margin, and madarosis, may occur in severe long-standing cases (**1**). **Atopic eczema (dermatitis)** is an occasional association. Flexural eczema is characterized by dry, lichenified or excoriated skin that may involve the elbow and knee flexures, ankles, and wrists (**A**).

2 and C

Posterior blepharitis is caused by meibomian gland dysfunction and alterations in meibomian gland secretions. Excessive and abnormal meibomian gland secretion manifests as capping of meibomian gland orifices with oil globules (**2**). **Acne rosacea** is a common association. It is characterized by erythema and papules involving the forehead, cheeks, and chin (**C**).

3 and B

Seborrhoeic blepharitis is characterized by hyperaemic and greasy anterior lid margins with sticking together of lashes (**3**). The scales are soft and located anywhere on the lid margin and lashes. **Seborrhoeic dermatitis** is a very common association. In young adults it typically affects the face whereas in elderly patients it may involve large areas of the body and even cause erythroderma (**B**).

What are these causes of heterochromia iridis?

1. Fuchs uveitis syndrome is a chronic anterior uveitis of insidious onset. It typically affects one eye of a young adult and frequently causes secondary cataract which may be the presenting feature. Heterochromia iridis is an important and common sign. Most frequently the affected eye is hypochromic. The nature of heterochromia is determined by the relative degrees of atrophy of the stroma and posterior pigment epithelium, as well as the patient's natural iris colour. In blue eyes, predominant stromal atrophy allows the posterior pigmented layer to show through and become the dominant pigmentation, so that the eye may become hyperchromic (reverse heterochromia).

2. Waardenburg syndrome is an AD condition characterized by hyperchromic heterochromia iridis, partial albinism, deafness, poliosis, white hair forelock, telecanthus, and synophrys or unusual facial hair distribution. Fundus pigment heterochromia may also be present.

3. Congenital Horner syndrome is characterized by ipsilateral hypochromic heterochromia, miosis, and mild ptosis. Heterochromia is not invariably present in congenital Horner syndrome, and rarely, it may occur in acquired Horner syndrome, even in adults.

4. Naevus of Ota is characterized by cutaneous and episcleral pigmentation. Ipsilateral hyperchromic heterochromia is common and may be associated with trabecular and fundus hyperpigmentation.

QUESTION 27

Match (1–3) with the gonioscopy (A–C)

1 and A

Aniridia is a rare bilateral congenital condition characterized by partial (**1**) or total loss of iris tissue. **Gonioscopy** even in eyes with 'total' aniridia usually shows a rudimentary frill of iris tissue (**A**). Glaucoma occurs in approximately 75% of patients and usually presents in late childhood or adolescence. It is caused by synechial angle closure secondary to the pulling forward of rudimentary iris tissue by contraction of pre-existing fibres that bridge the angle.

2 and C

Primary congenital glaucoma (PCG) is the most common of the congenital glaucomas. The clinical features depend on the age of onset and the level of IOP. Breaks in Descemet membrane secondary to corneal stretching may be associated with a sudden influx of aqueous into the corneal stroma. Haab striae represent healed breaks in Descemet membrane and appear as horizontal curvilinear lines (**2**). Impaired aqueous outflow in PCG is caused by maldevelopment of the angle (trabeculodysgenesis). **Gonioscopy** shows a flat iris insertion into the trabecular meshwork, absence of an angle recess, and translucent amorphous material (**C**).

3 and B

Axenfeld–Rieger syndrome is a spectrum of disorders designated in current nomenclature by the following eponyms: (a) *Axenfeld anomaly*, (b) *Rieger anomaly* and (c) *Rieger syndrome*. Axenfeld anomaly is characterized by posterior embryotoxon; **gonioscopy** shows strands of peripheral iris tissue attached to the cornea (**B**). In Rieger anomaly the iris attachments are broader and glaucoma occurs in 50% of cases. Rieger syndrome is associated with dental and facial anomalies.

QUESTION 28

What is the probable pathogen in each condition?

1. Angular blepharitis involves the lateral parts of the lids and is characterized by often unilateral red, scaly, macerated skin at the lateral or medial canthus. The infection is usually caused by ***Moraxella lacunata*** or ***S. aureus***.

2. Gonococcal conjunctivitis is characterized by intense conjunctival hyperaemia, chemosis, and profuse purulent discharge. Lymphadenopathy is prominent and, in severe cases, suppuration may occur. Corneal ulceration ensues if conjunctivitis is not treated appropriately.

3. Chronic canaliculitis is an uncommon condition, frequently caused by ***Actinomyces israelii*** (anaerobic Gram-positive bacteria). In most cases there is no identifiable predisposition. Concretions consisting of sulphur granules can be expressed on canalicular compression with a glass rod or they become evident following canaliculotomy.

4. Acute dacryocystitis is usually secondary to obstruction of the nasolacrimal duct. It causes a very tender, red, tense swelling at the medial canthus that may be associated with mild preseptal cellulitis. It is most commonly caused by ***S. aureus***.

5. Necrotizing fasciitis is an extremely rare rapidly progressive necrosis initially involving subcutaneous soft tissues and later the skin. It is usually caused by ***S. pyogenes***. Periocular infection is rare and may be secondary to trauma or surgery. It is characterized by black discoloration of skin due to gangrene secondary to underlying thrombosis. Unless treatment is prompt and appropriate death may result.

6. Ophthalmia neonatorum (neonatal conjunctivitis) develops within two weeks of birth as the result of infection transmitted from mother to infant during delivery. It is serious because of the lack of immunity in the infant and immaturity of the ocular surface (no lymphoid tissue and relatively poor tear film). **C. trachomatis** accounts for the majority of cases in developed countries and may also cause pneumonitis, otitis, and rhinitis.

What is this metabolic disease?

Amyloidosis is a term applied to a number of conditions of varying aetiology characterized by deposition of insoluble fibrillary protein in organs and tissues. Amyloid may be primary or secondary to chronic inflammatory disease, as well as systemic or local. The diagnosis is usually established by biopsy – Congo red stains amyloid orange-red (**1**). Involvement of the tongue giving rise to macroglossia is typical (**2**). Periorbital waxy plaques may be seen in primary amyloidosis (**3**). Ocular primary amyloidosis is seen in lattice corneal dystrophies types 1 and 3 (**4**), as conjunctival nodules (**5**), and with vitreous involvement that has a characteristic glasswool-like appearance (**6**). Lattice dystrophy type 2 is associated with systemic amyloidosis (Meretoja syndrome).

QUESTION 30

Which of these may give rise to cystoid macular oedema?

1. Retinal branch vein occlusion. FA shows blockage by blood and hypofluorescence due to retinal capillary non-perfusion. The most common cause of persistent poor visual acuity following branch vein occlusion is **CMO**. Some patients with visual acuity of 6/12 or worse may benefit from laser photocoagulation, provided the macula is oedematous rather than significantly ischaemic.

2. Retinitis pigmentosa. Late phase FA shows areas of bone-spicule hypofluorescence on a diffuse background of hyperfluorescence due to a window defect caused by atrophy of the RPE. **CMO** occurs in a minority of cases and may respond to systemic administration of acetazolamide.

3. Retinal periphlebitis is an inflammation of veins which may be primary, or secondary to a specific type of intraocular inflammatory process. FA shows irregular perivenous hyperfluorescence, some of which is patchy. **CMO** is a common cause of visual morbidity.

4. Retinal branch artery occlusion. FA shows delay in arterial filling and hypofluorescence of the involved segment due to blockage of background fluorescence by retinal swelling. Visual morbidity is caused by macular ischaemia and not oedema.

5. Background diabetic retinopathy. FA shows myriads of tiny hyperfluorescent dots, representing non-thrombosed microaneurysms and many scattered patches of hypofluorescence due to either blockage by haemorrhages or focal capillary non-perfusion. **CMO** is a common cause of visual impairment.

SECTION 1

ANSWERS

6. Soft drusen. FA shows late hyperfluorescent spots at the posterior due to staining. CMO does not occur in eyes with drusen, although they may subsequently lead to age-related macular degeneration.

epithelial oedema, microcyst formation, and bullous keratopathy (**A**). **Fuchs spot** is a slightly raised, pigmented lesion that may develop after a macular haemorrhage has absorbed (**B**). Fuchs also described heterochromic cyclitis.

QUESTION 31

Which three physicians described these conditions?

1. Henri Parinaud (1844–1905) was a French ophthalmologist. **Parinaud syndrome** is caused by a dorsal midbrain lesion, such as a pinealoma, resulting in vertical gaze palsy, convergence-retraction nystagmus, light-near dissociation with large pupils, and defective convergence (**A**). **Parinaud oculoglandular syndrome** is characterized by chronic fever, unilateral conjunctival granulomas with surrounding follicles (**B**), and prominent ipsilateral preauricular lymphadenopathy. By far most common cause is cat-scratch disease.

2. Alfred Vogt (1879–1943) was a Swiss ophthalmologist. **Vogt limbal girdle** is a common, innocuous age-related finding characterized by bilateral, narrow, crescentic white lesions running in the interpalpebral fissure along the nasal and temporal limbus (**A**). **Vogt striae** occur in keratoconus and are characterized by very fine, vertical, deep stromal striae (**B**), which disappear with external pressure on the globe. Vogt also described V–K–H syndrome and anterior crocodile shagreen.

3. Ernst Fuchs (1851–1930) was an Austrian ophthalmologist. **Fuchs endothelial dystrophy** is a bilateral disease in which there is accelerated corneal endothelial cell loss that eventually causes

QUESTION 32

Which pathogens are responsible for these conditions?

1. Rubella retinopathy is caused by transplacental transmission of virus to the fetus from an infected mother, usually during the first trimester of pregnancy. It is characterized by a 'salt and pepper' pigmentary disturbance involving the periphery and posterior pole. The prognosis is usually good although a small percentage of eyes may later develop choroidal neovascularization.

2. Acute retinal necrosis is a rare but devastating necrotizing retinitis that typically affects otherwise healthy individuals of all ages. It tends to be caused by herpes simplex in younger patients and herpes zoster in older individuals. It is characterized by peripheral retinal periarteritis associated with multifocal, deep, yellow-white, retinal infiltrates that gradually coalesce and progress to full-thickness retinal necrosis.

3. Neuroretinitis is characterized by papillitis and the subsequent development of a macular star figure composed of hard exudates. After several months visual acuity improves, with resolution of papillitis and then hard exudates – although initially the exudates may increase as disc swelling is resolving. A common cause of neuroretinitis is cat-scratch disease (benign lymphoreticulosis) which is caused by *Bartonella henselae* (a Gram-negative rod).

4. Cytomegalovirus retinitis is the most common ocular opportunistic infection among patients with AIDS. Fulminating retinitis is characterized by a dense, white, well-demarcated, geographical area of confluent opacification often associated with retinal haemorrhages that extends along the course of the retinal vascular arcades and may involve the optic nerve head.

5. Presumed ocular histoplasmosis represents an immunologic mediated response in individuals previously exposed to the *Histoplasma capsulatum* fungus. Inactive lesions consist of 'histo' spots consisting of atrophic, roundish lesions, often associated with pigment clumps within or at the margins of the scars. The lesions are scattered in the mid-retinal periphery and posterior fundus and are often associated with peripapillary atrophy which may be diffuse or focal.

6. *Pneumocystis carinii* choroiditis is caused by *P. carinii*, an opportunistic protozoan parasite, which is a major cause of morbidity and mortality in AIDS. It is characterized by flat, yellow, round, choroidal lesions, scattered throughout the posterior pole, which are frequently bilateral but cause little if any visual impairment. The presence of choroidal involvement is often a sign of extrapulmonary systemic dissemination and poor prognosis for life.

QUESTION 33

What are these associations of pigmentary retinopathy?

1. Oculodigital syndrome describes constant rubbing of the eyes by a blind child that may cause enophthalmos as a result of resorption of orbital fat. It is a feature of **Leber congenital amaurosis** which is an extremely serious AR retinal dystrophy and the commonest genetic cause of visual impairment in infants and children.

2. Refsum syndrome (heredopathia atactica polyneuritiformis) is an AR inborn error of metabolism due to a deficiency in the enzyme phytanic acid 2-hydroxylase resulting in the accumulation phytanic acid in the blood and body tissues. Clinical features include polyneuropathy, cerebellar ataxia, deafness, anosmia, cardiomyopathy, and ichthyosis. **Retinopathy** develops in the second decade and is characterized by generalized 'salt-and-pepper' changes.

3. Kearns–Sayre syndrome is a mitochondrial cytopathy associated with DNA deletions. Presentation is in the first to second decades with an insidious onset of bilateral and symmetrical ptosis, and limitation of ocular movements in all directions of gaze (progressive external ophthalmoplegia). **Retinopathy** is characterized by coarse pigment clumping which principally affects the central fundus.

4. Bardet–Biedl syndrome is an AR condition characterized by obesity, brachydactyly and polydactyly, dental anomalies, hypogenitalism, and renal disease. **Retinitis pigmentosa** is severe and almost 75% of patients are blind by the age of 20 years.

5. Usher syndrome is an AR condition which accounts for about 5% of all cases of profound deafness in children, and is responsible for about half of all cases of combined deafness and blindness. **Retinitis pigmentosa** develops before puberty.

6. Bassen–Kornzweig syndrome is an AR condition caused by deficiency in beta-lipoprotein resulting in intestinal malabsorption, spinocerebellar ataxia, ptosis and progressive external ophthalmoplegia. The blood film shows acanthocytosis in which erythrocytes have spiny surface projections. **Pigmentary retinopathy** develops towards the end of the first decade in which the pigment clumps are often larger than in classic retinitis pigmentosa and are not confined to the equatorial region.

QUESTION 34

Match the eyelid tumour (1–3) with the histology (A–C)

1 and B

Sebaceous gland carcinoma is a very rare slow-growing tumour which most frequently affects the elderly. It usually arises from the meibomian glands, although on occasion it may arise from the glands of Zeis or sebaceous glands in the caruncle. It most commonly involves the upper eyelid, where meibomian glands are more numerous (**1**). **Histology** shows lobules of cells with pale foamy vacuolated cytoplasm and large hyperchromatic nuclei that stain positive (red) for lipid (**B**).

2 and A

Basal cell carcinoma (BCC) is by far the most common malignant eyelid tumour. It most frequently arises from the lower eyelid, followed in relative frequency by the medial canthus, upper eyelid, and lateral canthus. (**2**). **Histology** shows downward proliferation of basal cells that may exhibit palisading at the periphery of a lobule of cells (**A**).

3 and C

Keratoacanthoma is a rare tumour which usually occurs in fair-skinned individuals with a history of chronic sun exposure. It is found more frequently than would be expected by chance in patients on immunosuppressive therapy following renal transplants. The tumour grows rapidly and then involutes slowly. During the period of regression the central part of the lesion becomes hyperkeratotic and a keratin-filled crater may develop (**3**). **Histology** shows irregular thickened epidermis surrounded by acanthotic squamous epithelium. The sharp transition from the thickened to normal adjacent epidermis is referred to as shoulder formation. A keratin-filled crater may be seen (**C**). Histopathologically, keratoacanthoma is regarded as part of the spectrum of squamous cell carcinoma into which it may evolve.

QUESTION 35

Match 1 with the skin rash (A–D)

1 and C

Lyme disease (borreliosis) is an infection caused by a flagellated spirochaete, *Borrelia burgdorferi*, transmitted through the bite of a hard shelled tick (**1**) of the genus *Ixodes* which feeds on a variety of large mammals, particularly deer. Several days after the bite, a pathognomonic annular expanding skin lesion (**erythema chronicum migrans** – **C**) develops, which may be accompanied by constitutional symptoms, and lymphadenopathy. Protective clothing and insect repellents should be used in tick-infested areas.

A. 'Target' lesions have a red centre surrounded by a pale area, in turn encircled by an erythematous ring. They occur in **Stevens–Johnson syndrome** – a mucocutaneous blistering disease thought to be either a delayed hypersensitivity response to drugs or to epithelial cell antigens modified by drug exposure.

B. Necrobiosis lipoidica describes waxy plaques with irregular margins and shiny centres that involve the shins of a small minority of patients with **diabetes**.

D. Erythema nodosum is characterized by tender erythematous plaques that typically involve the knees and shins, and occasionally the thighs and forearms. Important associations include **sarcoidosis**, TB, and inflammatory bowel disease; about 20% of cases are idiopathic.

QUESTION 36

Match the gonioscopy (1–3) with the pathology (A–C)

I and B

Secondary inflammatory glaucoma frequently presents a diagnostic and therapeutic challenge. The pathogenesis of elevation of IOP may be uncertain and multiple mechanisms involved. Angle-closure without pupil block occurs in chronic anterior uveitis and is the result of deposition of inflammatory cells and debris in the angle (**1** and **B**). Subsequent organization and contraction of debris pulls the peripheral iris over the trabeculum, resulting in gradual progressive synechial angle closure and eventual elevation of IOP.

2 and A

Secondary trabecular block glaucoma. Approximately 5% of eyes with intraocular tumours develop a secondary elevation of IOP due to several possible mechanisms. Trabecular block may be caused by infiltration of the trabeculum by neoplastic cells originating from an iris melanoma (**2** and **A**), or occasionally by trabecular blockage by macrophages which have injected pigment and tumour cells

(melanomalytic glaucoma), by a mechanism similar to that in phacolytic glaucoma.

3 and C

Neovascular glaucoma is a serious condition which occurs as a result of iris neovascularization (rubeosis iridis) secondary to severe, diffuse and chronic retinal ischaemia. The angle becomes progressively closed by contraction of fibrovascular tissue which pulls the peripheral iris over the trabeculum (**3**). The angle becomes closed circumferentially in a zipper-like fashion (**C**) resulting in very high IOP, severe visual impairment, congestion of the globe, and pain.

QUESTION 37

What do these red reflexes show?

1. Lens subluxation may be caused by severe blunt trauma that tears the zonules. The lens tends to deviate towards the meridian of the intact zonules. The edge of the subluxated lens is usually visible with mydriasis, and the iris may tremble on ocular movement.

2. Vossius ring consists of iris pigment imprint on the anterior lens capsule which corresponds to the size of the miosed pupil. It may be caused by blunt ocular trauma or following dilatation of the pupil in eyes with posterior synechiae.

3. Posterior capsular opacification is a common problem following cataract surgery. Elschnig pearls are caused by the proliferation and migration of residual equatorial epithelial cells along the posterior capsular surface at the site of apposition between the remnants of the anterior and posterior capsule.

4. Lamellar cataract affects a particular lamella of the lens both anteriorly and posteriorly and in some cases is associated with radial extensions (riders). It is usually AD and occurs in isolation.

5. Megalocornea is a rare, XLR, bilateral condition in which the corneal diameter is 13 mm or more and the anterior chamber is very deep. Corrected visual acuity is good despite high myopia and astigmatism. It is associated with pigment dispersion but normal intraocular pressure.

6. Keratoconus is a progressive disorder in which the cornea assumes a conical shape secondary to stromal thinning and protrusion. In early cases direct ophthalmoscopy from a distance of one foot (30 cm) shows an 'oil droplet' reflex. Retinoscopy shows an irregular 'scissor' reflex.

QUESTION 38

Match the face (1–3) with the fundus (A–C)

1 and C

Stickler syndrome (hereditary arthro-ophthalmopathy) is an AD disorder of collagen connective tissue, resulting in abnormal vitreous, myopia, and a variable degree of orofacial abnormality, deafness, and arthropathy. Facial anomalies include a flat nasal bridge and maxillary hypoplasia (**1**). Stickler syndrome is the commonest inherited cause of retinal detachment in children. It develops in approximately 30% of cases in the first decade of life, often as a result of multiple or giant tears that may involve both eyes. Because the prognosis is poor, patients should be examined regularly and retinal breaks treated prophylactically. The vitreous shows characteristic liquefaction (empty vitreous) and circumferential

membranes (**C**). The peripheral retina shows atypical radial lattice degeneration.

2 and B

Tuberous sclerosis (Bourneville disease) is an AD phacomatosis characterized by hamartomas in multiple organ systems. The classic triad comprises (a) *epilepsy*, (b) *mental retardation* and (c) *adenoma sebaceum*. The latter is universal and consists of fibroangiomatous red papules with a butterfly distribution around the nose and cheeks (**2**). About 50% of patients with tuberous sclerosis have fundus astrocytomas which may be multiple (**B**) and bilateral.

3 and A

Sturge–Weber syndrome (encephalotrigeminal angiomatosis) is a sporadic phacomatosis. Trisystem disease involves the face, leptomeninges, and eyes, and bisystem disease involves the face and eyes or the face and leptomeninges. Facial naevus flammeus (port-wine stain), extending over the area corresponding to the distribution of one or more branches of the trigeminal nerve is universal (**3**). Some patients have ipsilateral diffuse choroidal haemangioma characterized by a deep red 'tomato-ketchup' colour most marked at the posterior pole (**A**). Other ocular features include ipsilateral glaucoma, episcleral haemangioma, and rarely, iris heterochromia.

QUESTION 39

Which of (A–D) is not associated with 1?

C Cataract

Prematurity (**1**) may be associated with the following. **Retinopathy of prematurity** (ROP) is a proliferative retinopathy affecting premature infants of low birth weight, who have been exposed to high ambient oxygen concentrations. Stage 3 ROP is characterized by a ridge and extraretinal neovascularization (**A**). **Strabismus** (**B**) has an increased prevalence in preterm birth. **Myopia** (**D**) is a consequence of low birth weight, even in the absence of (ROP) (myopia of prematurity), and is also a complication of severe ROP. Myopia of prematurity has its onset during school years, whereas that associated with ROP begins in infancy.

QUESTION 40

Which is the odd one out?

4 Anterior uveitis

Sjögren syndrome is characterized by autoimmune inflammation and destruction of lacrimal and salivary glands. The condition is classified as primary when it exists in isolation, and secondary when associated with other diseases such as rheumatoid arthritis, SLE, systemic sclerosis, primary biliary cirrhosis, chronic active hepatitis, and myasthenia gravis. Primary Sjögren syndrome affects females more commonly than males. It is characterized by enlargement of salivary glands (**1**), and occasionally lacrimal glands (**2**), and a dry mouth and a dry tongue (**3**). Biopsy of lacrimal or salivary glands shows disruption of normal tubuloacinar architecture by a dense lymphocytic infiltrate surrounding dilated epithelial ducts (**5**). Deficiency of lacrimal secretion gives rise to keratoconjunctivitis sicca and filamentary keratitis (**6**).

QUESTION 41

What multiple pathology is present in these conditions?

1. Angioid streaks and **choroidal neovascularization.** Late phase FA shows linear hyperfluorescence due to RPE window defects emanating from the disc, and a round area of hyperfluorescence at the macula due to staining of a choroidal neovascular membrane. Eyes with angioid streaks may also lose vision due to foveal involvement by a streak or choroidal rupture and haemorrhage caused by blunt ocular trauma.

2. Combined anterior ischaemic optic neuropathy and **cilioretinal artery occlusion** typically affects elderly patients with giant cell arteritis and carries a very poor prognosis. The optic disc is elevated and pale and the macula shows pallor due to ischaemia. A cilioretinal artery, present in 20% of the population, arises from the posterior ciliary circulation and supplies the macula and papillomacular bundle.

3. Congenital optic disc pit and **coloboma** is an extremely rare combination. The pit occupies the temporal part of a small disc and the coloboma is located inferiorly.

4. Iris tumour and an **anterior chamber intraocular lens.**

5. OCT shows **cystoid macular oedema** and **retinal pigment epithelial detachment.**

6. Thyroid ophthalmopathy and **vitiligo.** There is bilateral proptosis and lid retraction, and left exotropia. Vitiligo is characterized by sharply-defined white macules due to absence of melanocytes. It is associated with thyrotoxicosis as well as other autoimmune diseases such as diabetes, pernicious anaemia, and adrenal disease.

QUESTION 42

What treatment has caused these complications?

1. Cataract following long-term use of topical steroids for limbal vernal disease. Limbal vernal disease typically affects black and Asian patients who develop gelatinous papillae on the limbal conjunctiva that may be associated with discrete white spots at their apices (Trantas dots). If possible long-term use of topical steroids should be avoided as it may cause cataract, and elevation of intraocular pressure in susceptible individuals.

2. Scleral thinning due to topical mitomycin C used to prevent recurrence following excision of pterygium. In most cases recurrences can be prevented without mitomycin C by using the appropriate surgical technique.

3. Cataract following intravitreal injection of silicone oil for treatment of complex retinal detachment. The emulsified silicone oil has migrated superiorly in the anterior chamber (inverted 'pseudo-hypopyon').

4. Surgically-induced scleritis following scleral buckling. Scleritis may also be induced by other procedures such as squint surgery and trabeculectomy. It typically starts within 3 weeks of the surgical procedure.

5. Corneal precipitation of ciprofloxacin following topical treatment of bacterial keratitis may impede healing.

6. Thin cystic drainage bleb following the use of adjuvant antimetabolites. Adjunctive antimetabolites are used to enhance the success rate of trabeculectomy, particularly in difficult cases. Problems include chronic hypotony, late-onset-bleb leak, and endophthalmitis.

QUESTION 43

What do these red-free images show?

1. Macular pseudohole which is caused by a defect in an epiretinal membrane.

2. Serous macular detachment associated with congenital optic disc pit develops in about 45% of eyes with non-central pits. Initially, there is a schisis-like separation of the inner layers of the retina which communicates with the pit. This is followed by serous detachment of the outer retinal layers which may be associated with subretinal deposits. This appearance may be mistaken for central serous retinopathy.

3. Fundus flavimaculatus is an AR retinal dystrophy that presents in adult life characterized by bilateral, ill-defined, yellow-white retinal flecks that may show autofluorescence. The prognosis is relatively good and patients may remain asymptomatic for many years unless a fleck involves the fovea or geographic atrophy develops.

4. Anterior ischaemic optic neuropathy is the result of partial or total infarction of the optic nerve head caused by occlusion of the short posterior ciliary arteries. The two main types are arteritic (caused by giant cell arteritis) and non-arteritic. Fundus examination shows disc pallor associated with diffuse or sectoral oedema often with a few peripapillary splinter-shaped haemorrhages.

5. Superotemporal retinal nerve fibre bundle defect. In primary open-angle glaucoma subtle retinal nerve fibre layer defects precede the development of detectable optic disc and visual field changes.

Retinal nerve fibre dropout may be diffuse or localized. Localized damage is characterized by slit defects in the retinal nerve fibre layer which is best visualized with a green filter. As glaucomatous damage progresses the defects become larger.

6. Opaque nerve fibres are white feathery streaks running within the retinal nerve fibre layer towards the disc. Only one eye is affected in the vast majority of cases. Ocular associations of extensive nerve fibre myelination include high myopia, anisometropia, and amblyopia. Systemic associations include neurofibromatosis-1 and Gorlin (multiple basal cell naevus) syndrome.

QUESTION 44

Match the anterior segment (1–3) with the fundus (A–C)

I and C

Anterior lenticonus is a congenital bilateral axial projection of the anterior lens surface (**1**). About 90% of patients have Alport syndrome which is an XLD condition characterized by chronic renal disease and deafness. Patients also exhibit scattered, yellowish, **punctate perimacular flecks** (**C**).

2 and B

Aniridia is a rare, congenital, sporadic or hereditary, bilateral, total (**2**) or partial absence of the iris. The fundus may show **foveal hypoplasia** (**B**), optic nerve hypoplasia, and occasionally choroidal colobomas. Sporadic aniridia (AN-2) carries a 30% risk of Wilm tumour developing before the age of 5 years.

3 and A

Rubeosis iridis refers to neovascularization of the iris (**3**) which, if advanced, causes intractable sec-ondary angle-closure glaucoma. Rubeosis occurs as a response to severe, diffuse and chronic retinal ischaemia, most frequently associated with **ischaemic central retinal vein occlusion** (**A**).

QUESTION 45

Match the systemic feature (1–3) with the cornea (A–C)

I and A

Fabry disease (alpha galactosidase deficiency) is an XL metabolic disease that causes a chronic progressive painful small-fibre neuropathy, renal disease, heart disease, and stroke. The skin shows characteristic purple telangiectasis (**angiokeratoma corporis diffusum**) in the lower abdomen (**1**). **Vortex keratopathy** (**A**) is universal. Other ocular features include lens opacities, conjunctival telangiectasis, retinal vascular tortuosity, third nerve palsy, and nystagmus.

2 and C

Familial hypercholesterolaemia is caused by a reduction or absence of functional low-density-lipoprotein (LDL) receptors due to a defect in the LDL receptor gene. Excessive tissue deposits may cause **xanthomata** in the extensor tendons over tissue points (**2**) and **corneal arcus** (**C**).

3 and B

The mucopolysaccharidoses (MPS) comprise a group of inherited deficiencies of catabolic glycosidase necessary for hydrolysis of mucopolysaccharides. Inheritance is AR except with the two subtypes of Hunter syndrome which are XLR. Systemic features, which vary with the type of MPS, include **facial coarseness** (**3**), skeletal anomalies, mental retardation, and heart disease. **Diffuse stromal**

corneal clouding (**B**) occurs in all MPS except Hunter and Sanfilippo. In Hurler and Scheie syndromes corneal deposits are most severe and present at birth. Corneal clouding in this setting should be differentiated from that associated with congenital glaucoma, rubella, congenital hereditary endothelial dystrophy, and birth trauma.

QUESTION 46

Who invented these operations?

1. Anthony Molteno, a South African ophthalmologist, invented the artificial glaucoma drainage implant in 1969. The device creates a communication between the anterior chamber and subconjunctival space. It is used mainly in cases that have either failed or are unsuitable for conventional drainage surgery.

2. Charles Kelman, an American ophthalmologist, described phacoemulsification in 1967.

3. Robert Machemer, a German ophthalmologist working in America, described pars plana vitrectomy in 1971.

4. Tadeusz Krwawicz, a Polish ophthalmologist, described intracapsular cataract extraction by cryoadhesion in 1961.

5. Sir Harold Ridley, an English ophthalmologist, performed the first intraocular lens implantation in 1949.

6. Harvey Lincoff, an American ophthalmologist, described local scleral buckling with a sponge explant in 1965. Until then most retinal detachment procedures involved encirclement.

QUESTION 47

Match the orbital disorder (1–3) with the CT (A–C)

I and B

Preseptal cellulitis is characterized by unilateral, periorbital oedema that is red and tender (**1**). **Coronal CT** shows opacification anterior to the orbital septum and lack of involvement of orbital tissue (**B**). Unlike orbital cellulitis, proptosis and chemosis are absent, and visual acuity, papillary reactions, and ocular motility are unimpaired.

2 and A

Thyroid ophthalmopathy manifests bilateral axial proptosis and asymmetrical lid retraction (**2**). **Axial CT** shows bilateral enlargement of extraocular muscles except the lateral recti (**A**). The most common ocular mobility defect is impairment of elevation due to fibrotic contraction of the inferior rectus.

3 and C

Benign lacrimal gland tumour causes fullness in the lacrimal gland fossa and inferior displacement of the globe (**3**). **Coronal CT** shows a lesion in the superior orbit without bony erosion (**C**). Treatment involves complete excision without preliminary biopsy so as not to cause seeding of the tumour.

QUESTION 48

What are these colour vision tests?

1. Ishihara test is used mainly to screen for congenital protan and deuteran defects. It consists of a test plate followed by 16 plates each with a matrix of dots arranged to show a central shape or number which the subject is asked to identify. A colour deficient person will only be able to identify some of the figures. Inability to identify the test plate (provided visual acuity is sufficient) indicates malingering.

2. Farnsworth–Munsell 100-hue is the most sensitive for both congenital and acquired colour defects but is seldom used in practice. Despite the name it consists of 85 hue caps contained in four separate racks in each of which the two end caps are fixed while the others are loose so they can be randomized by the examiner.

3. Hardy–Rand–Rittler is similar to Ishihara but more sensitive since it can detect all three congenital defects.

4. City University test consists of ten plates each containing a central colour and four peripheral colours. The subject selects the peripheral colour which most closely matches the central.

together with a large triangle of redundant skin. It is used in cases of marked generalized involutional ectropion with excess skin.

3. Tenzel flap is used to aid closure of a moderate-size lid defect following resection of a malignant lower lid tumour.

4. Mustarde cheek rotation flap is used to aid closure of a large lower lid defect following removal of a malignant lower lid tumour. It requires reconstruction of the posterior lamella.

5. Wies procedure is used to treat involutional entropion. It consists of full-thickness horizontal lid-splitting and insertion of everting sutures. The scar creates a barrier between the preseptal and pretarsal orbicularis, and the everting suture transfers the pull of the lower lid retractors from the tarsus to the skin and orbicularis.

QUESTION 49

What are these eponymous eyelid procedures?

1. Fasanella–Servat procedure involves excision of the upper border of the tarsus together with the lower border of Muller muscle and conjunctiva. It may be used in cases of mild ptosis with levator function of at least 10 mm. This includes most cases of Horner syndrome and very mild congenital ptosis. This procedure is now seldom performed by experts who prefer to excise Muller muscle and overlying conjunctiva and reattach the resected edges.

2. Kuhnt–Szymanowski procedure involves excision of a pentagon of full-thickness lid laterally

QUESTION 50

What are these signs?

1. Munson sign is a bulging of the lower lid on down-gaze in keratoconus.

2. Dalrymple sign manifests lid retraction with the eyes in the primary position.

3. von Graefe sign is retarded descent of the upper lid on down-gaze.

4. Bell phenomenon describes upward rolling of the eye on attempted lid closure.

5. Hutchinson sign describes a rash involving the tip and side of the nose in herpes zoster ophthalmicus resulting from involvement of the external nasal nerve which is the terminal branch of the nasociliary nerve. It correlates significantly with the subsequent development of ocular complications.

6. Setting sun sign describes downward displacement of the eyes so that they resemble a sun setting beneath the lower lids. Causes include increased intracranial pressure, hydrocephalus, and a pineal tumour.

Section 2

Questions 51 to 100. Answers start on page 130.

Q 51 What are these malignancies?

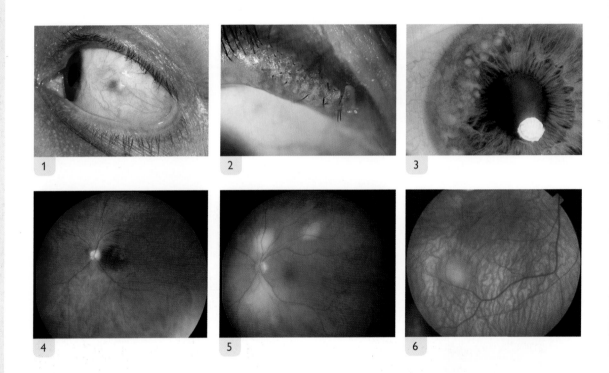

Answer on page 130

Q **52** Match the eyelash disorders (1–3) with the aetiology (A–C)

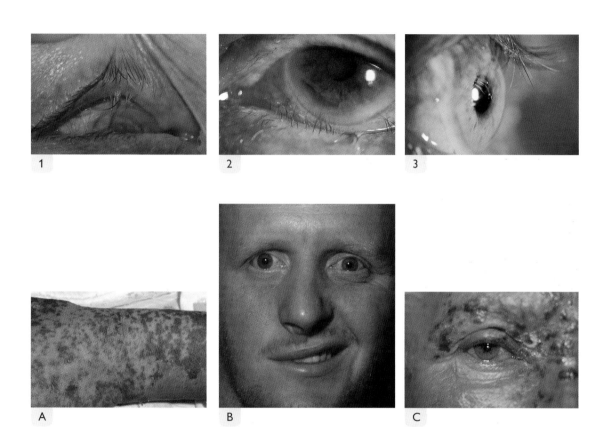

1

2

3

A

B

C

Answer on pages 130–131

Q **53** What are these items?

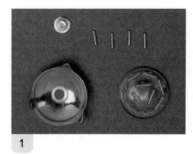

1

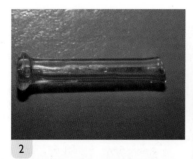

2

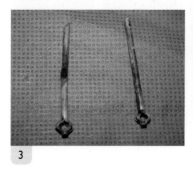

3

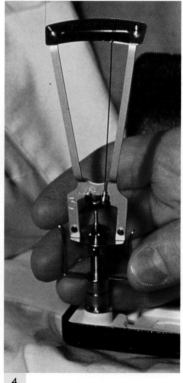

4

Answer on page 131

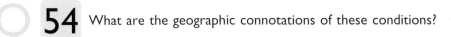

Q **54** What are the geographic connotations of these conditions?

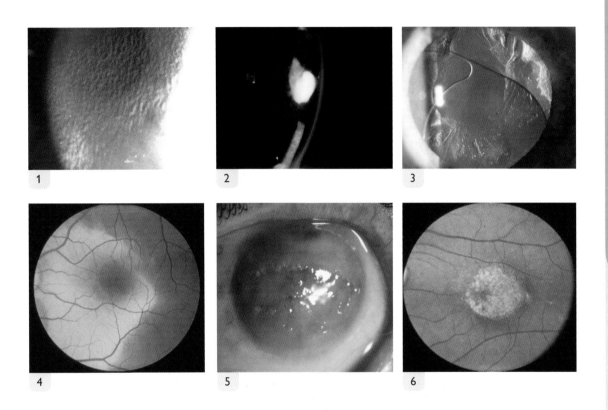

Answer on pages 131–132

SECTION 1

SECTION 2

SECTION 3

SECTION 4

Q 55 End-stage disease of which conditions?

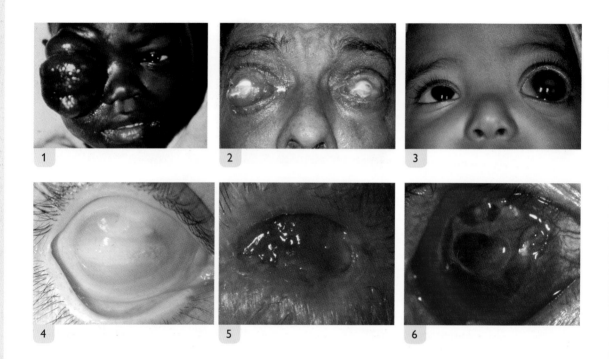

Answer on page 132

Q 56 What treatment has been performed?

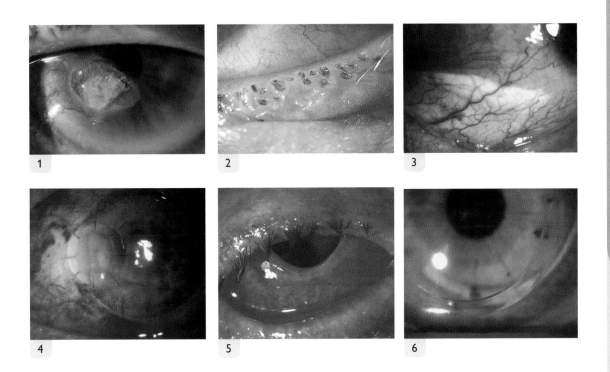

1

2

3

4

5

6

Answer on page 132

Q 57 What has caused these superior tarsal lesions?

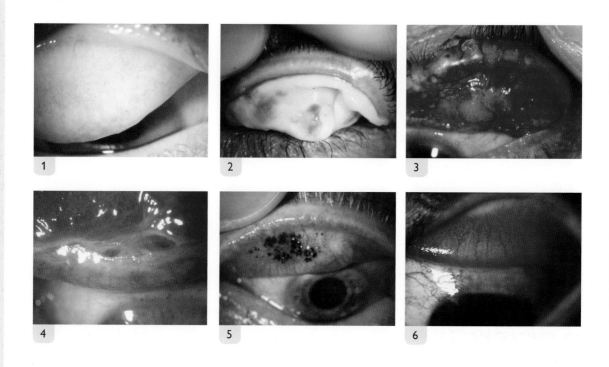

1 2 3

4 5 6

Answer on pages 132–133

Q **58** What is this systemic disease?

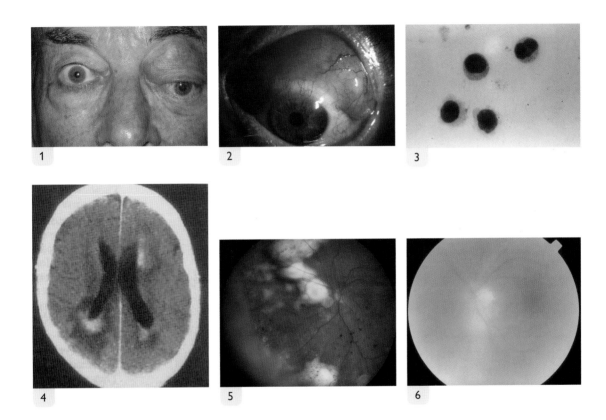

1

2

3

4

5

6

Answer on page 133

Q **59** What types of ptosis are shown?

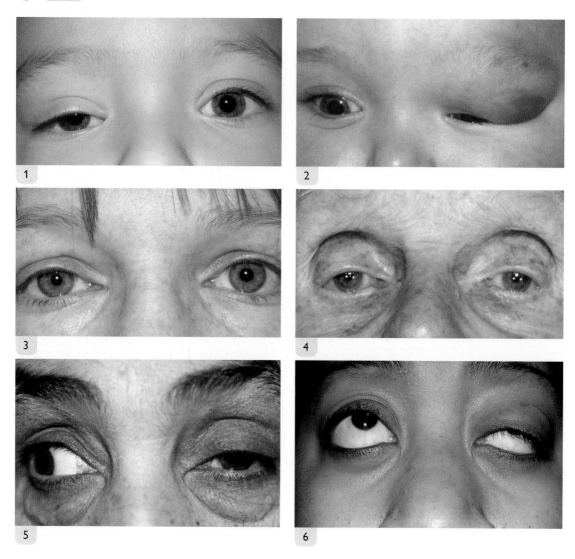

Answer on pages 133–134

Q **60** What are these orthoptic instruments?

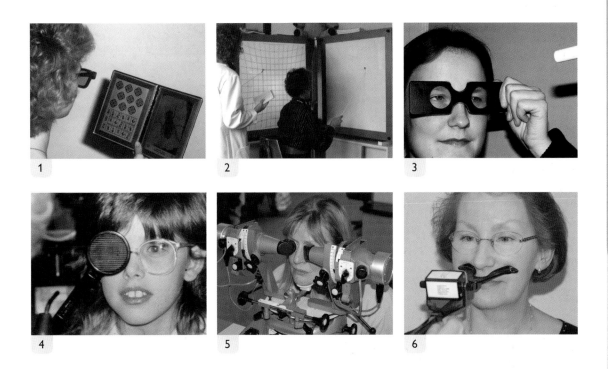

1

2

3

4

5

6

Answer on pages 134–135

Q 61 Match the fundus (1–3) with the scan (A–C)

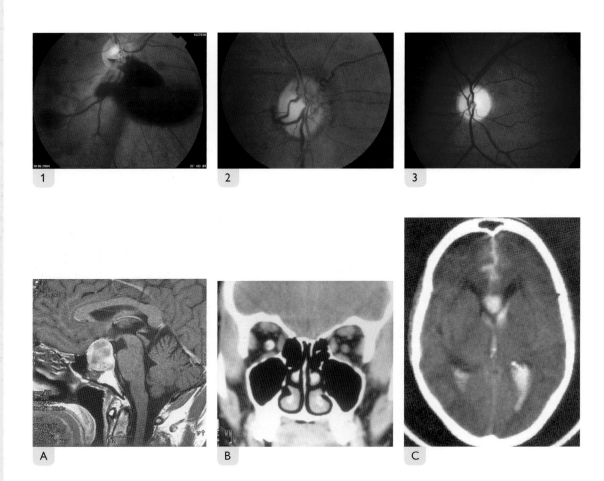

Answer on page 135

Q **62** What are these signs?

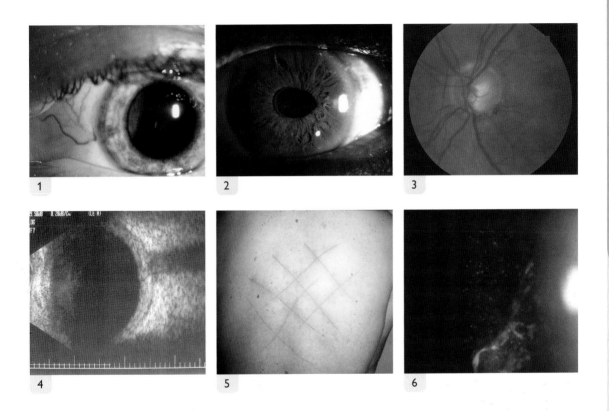

Answer on page 135

63 What are these complications of intraocular lens implantation?

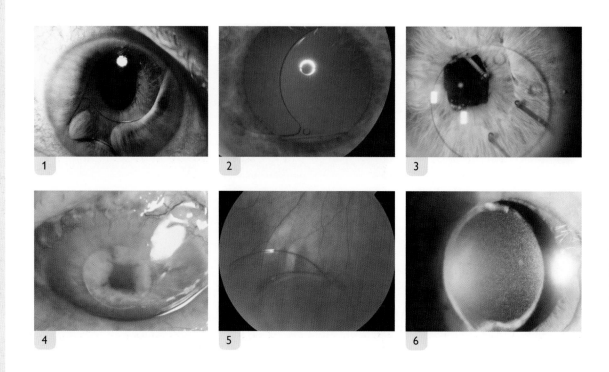

Answer on pages 135–136

Q **64** What are these subtle conditions?

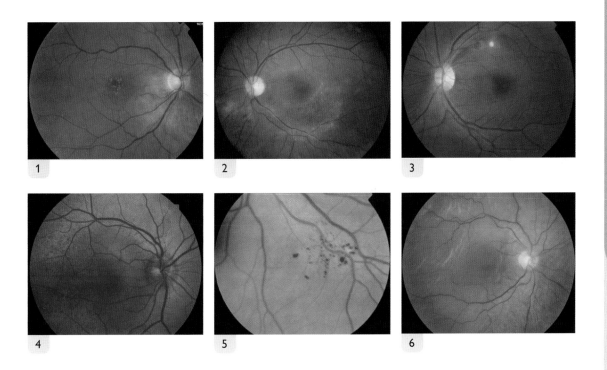

Answer on page 136

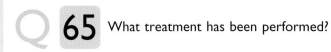

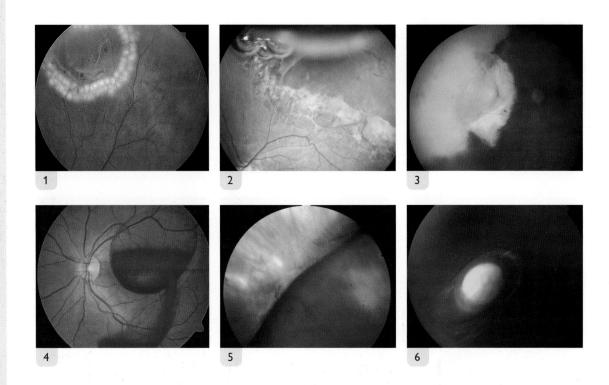

Answer on pages 136–137

Q 66 Who invented?

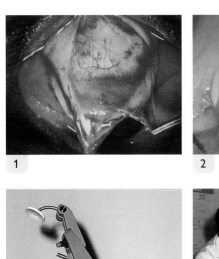

1

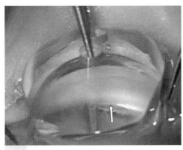

2

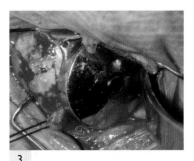

3

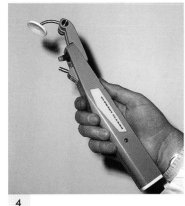

4

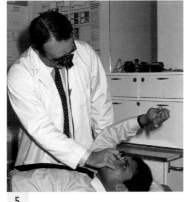

5

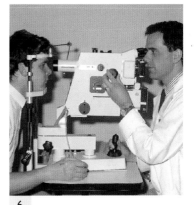

6

Answer on page 137

Q **67** Match the conjunctival lesion (1–3) with the histology (A–C)

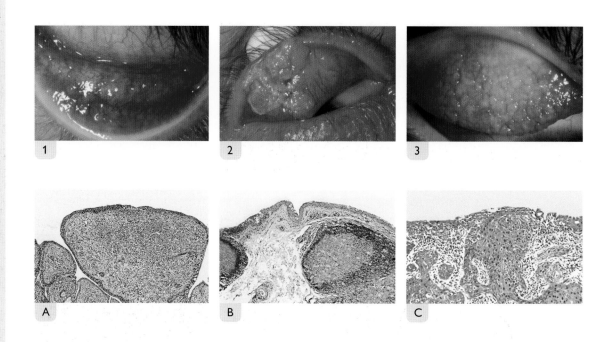

Answer on page 138

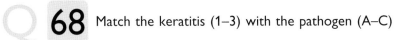

Q 68   Match the keratitis (1–3) with the pathogen (A–C)

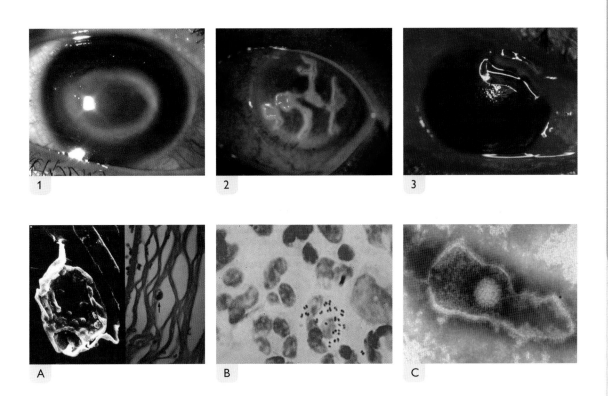

Answer on page 138

Q 69 What are these neuroimaging techniques?

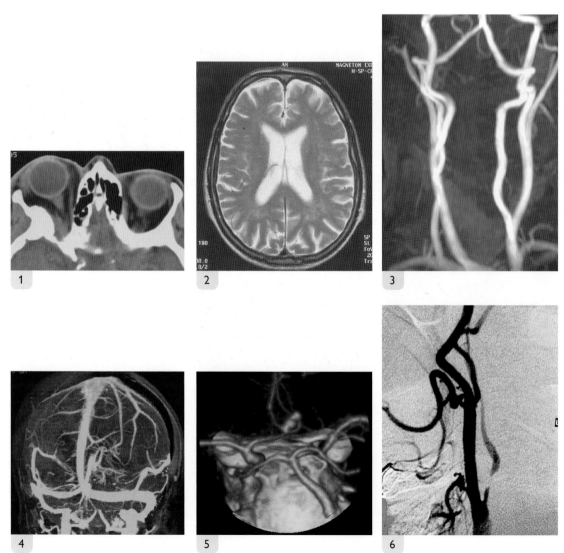

Answer on pages 138–139

Q **70** Match the lashes (1–3) with the skin (A–C)

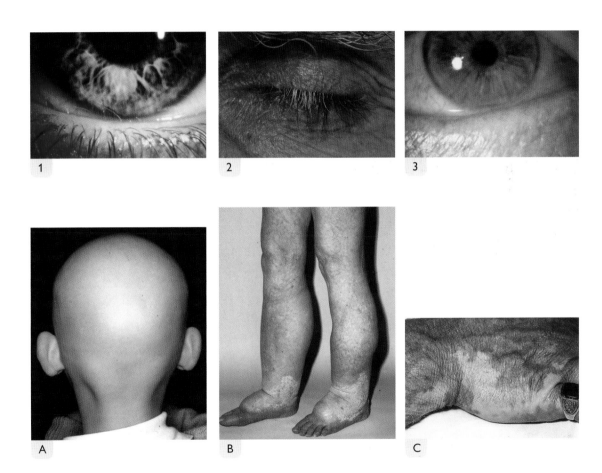

1

2

3

A

B

C

Answer on pages 139–140

Q 71 Toxoplasmosis or toxocariasis?

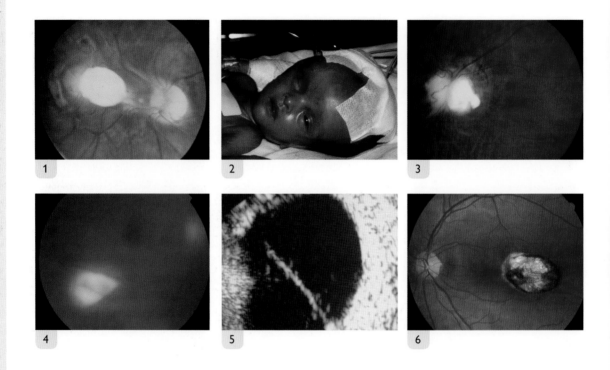

Answer on page 140

What are the underlying causes of the hard exudates?

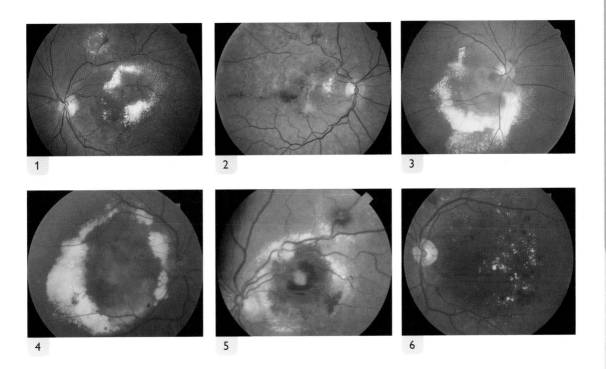

Answer on pages 140–141

Q 73 What are these instruments?

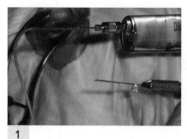

1

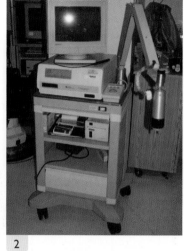

2

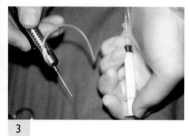

3

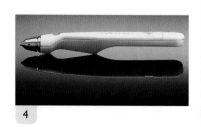

4

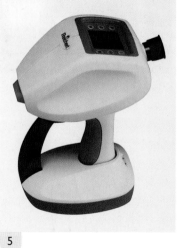

5

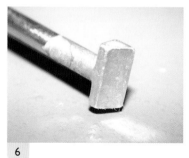

6

Answer on page 141

Q 74 What are these subtle lesions?

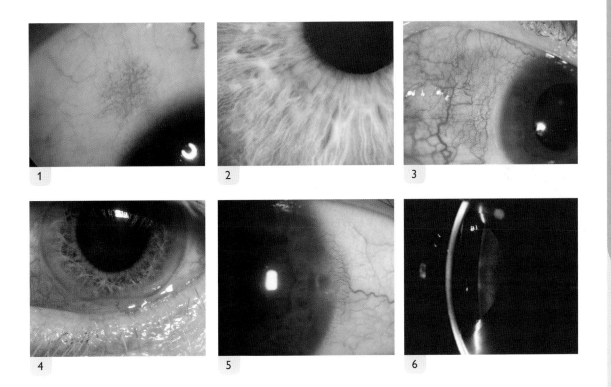

1

2

3

4

5

6

Answer on pages 141–142

Q 75 Match the mouth (1–3) with the eye (A–C)

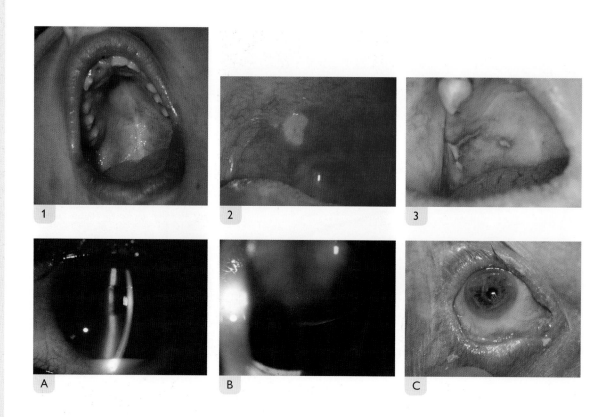

Answer on page 142

Q **76** Match the eye (1–3) with the treatment (A–C)

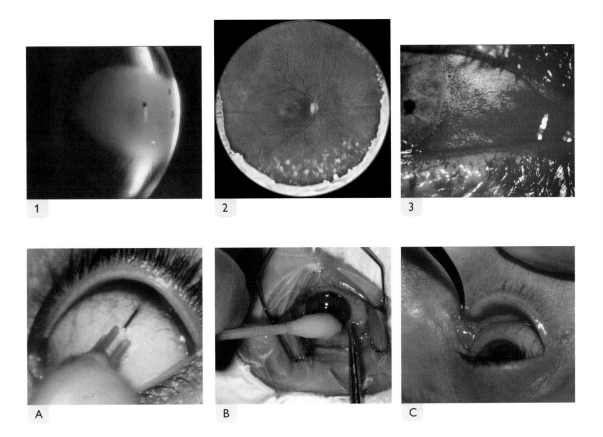

Answer on page 143

Q 77 What has caused these iris transillumination defects?

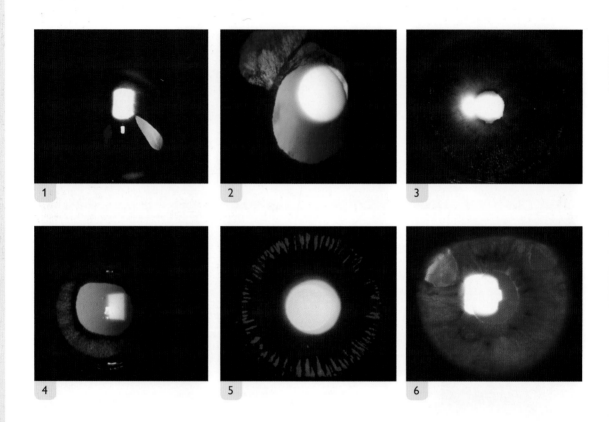

Answer on pages 143–144

Q 78 What have these conditions in common?

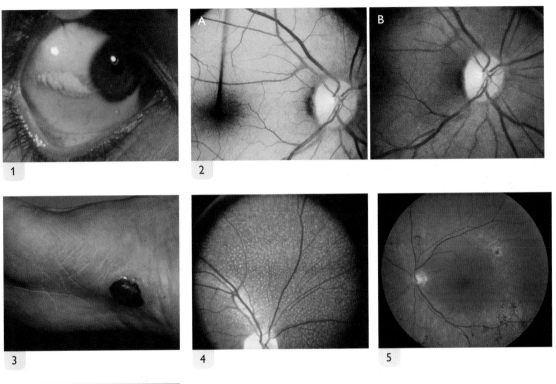

1

A

2

B

3

4

5

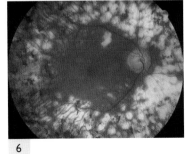

6

Answer on page 144

Q 79 What are these causes of leukocoria?

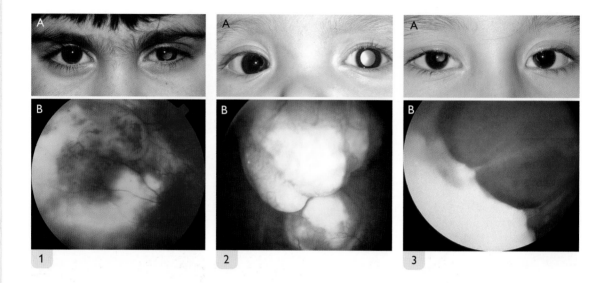

Answer on page 145

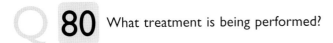

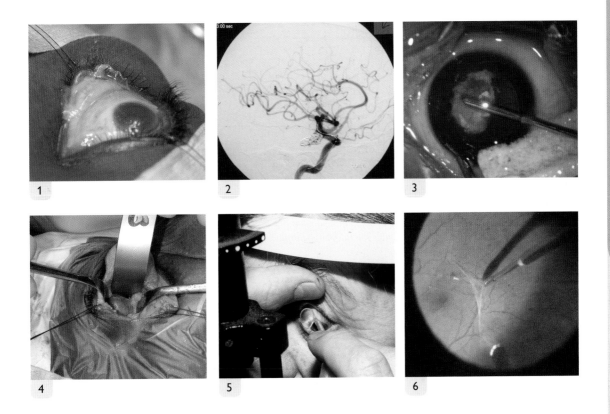

Answer on pages 145–146

81 Which ophthalmologists described these?

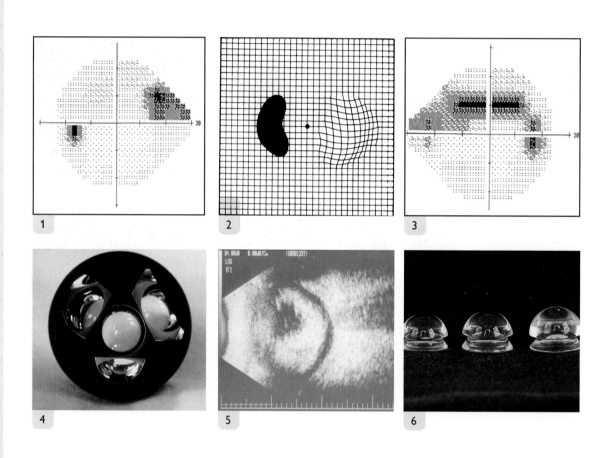

Answer on page 146

Q 82 Benign or malignant eyelid lesions?

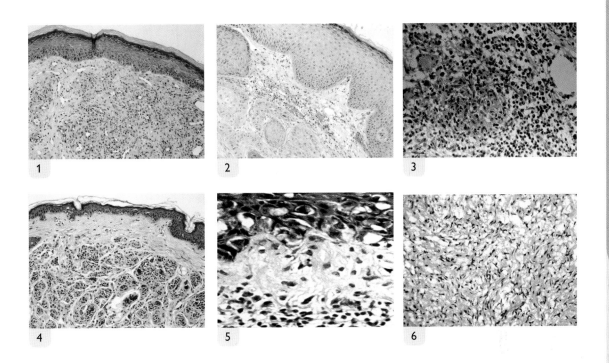

Answer on pages 146–147

111

Q **83** Which is the odd one out?

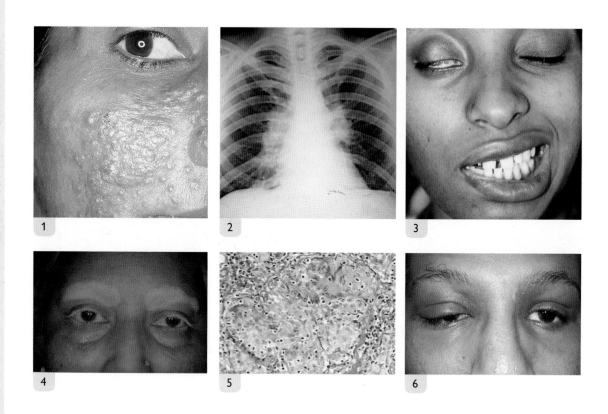

1

2

3

4

5

6

Answer on page 147

Q 84 What are these juxtalimbal lesions?

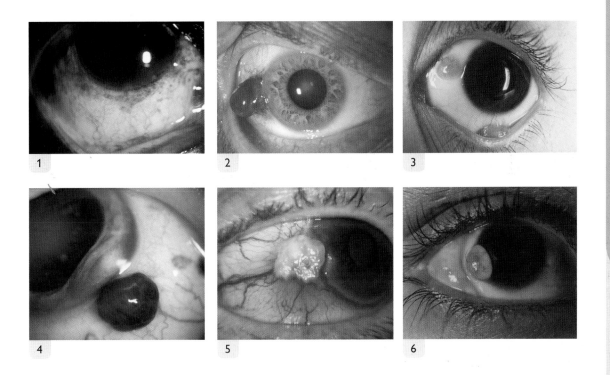

Answer on pages 147–148

Q **85** What are these?

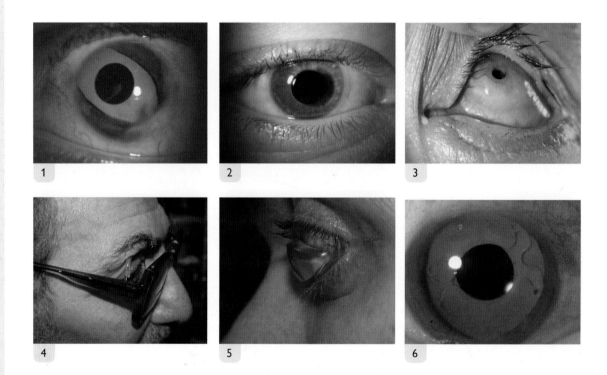

Answer on page 148

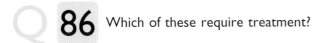

Which of these require treatment?

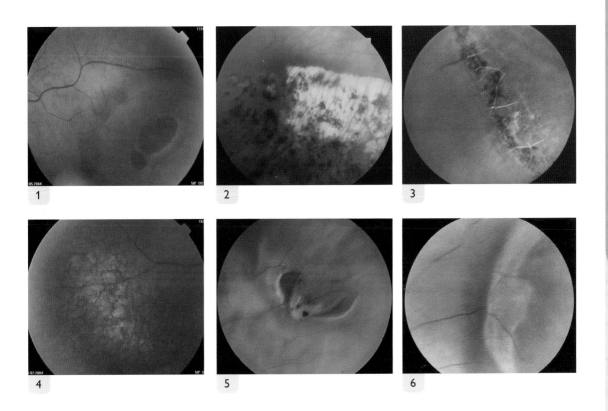

1

2

3

4

5

6

Answer on page 148

Q 87 What procedures were responsible for these complications?

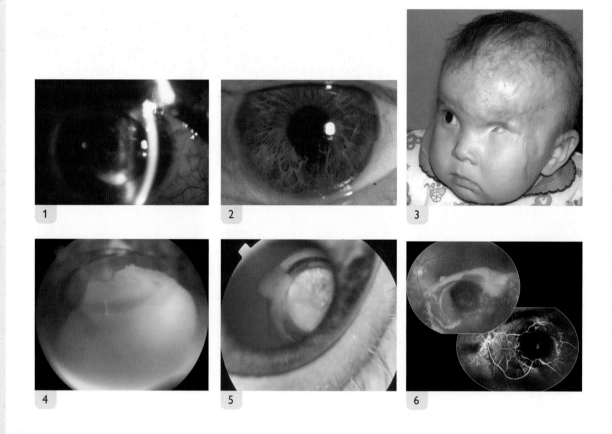

Answer on pages 148–149

Q **88** Match the angiogram (1–3) with the OCT (A–C)

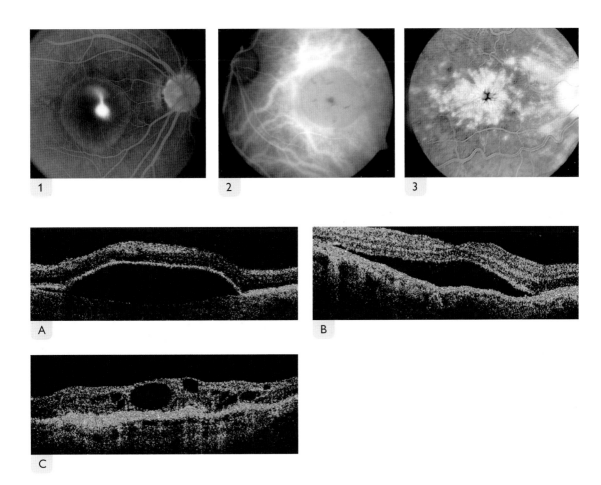

Answer on page 149

Q 89 What are the underlying causes of the cotton-wool spots?

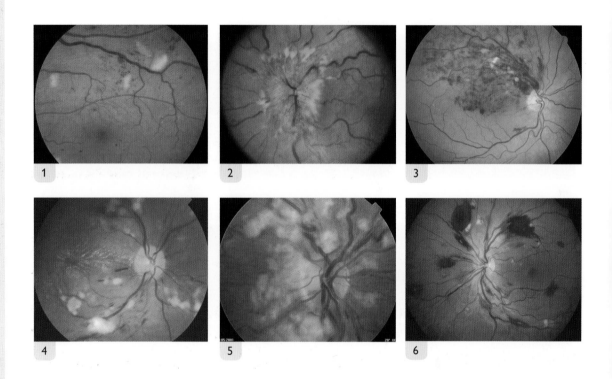

Answer on pages 149–150

90 What are these complications of penetrating keratoplasty?

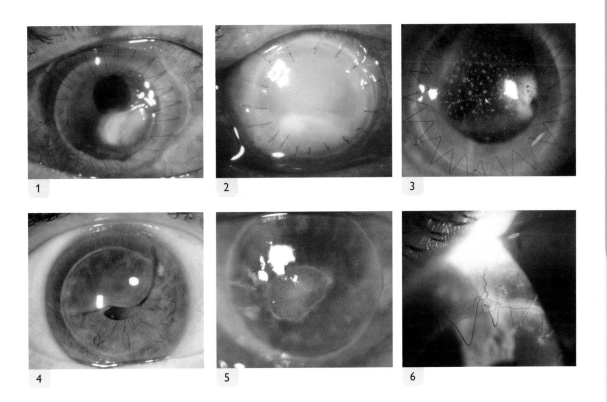

1

2

3

4

5

6

Answer on pages 150–151

Q **91**
What are these ocular imaging techniques?

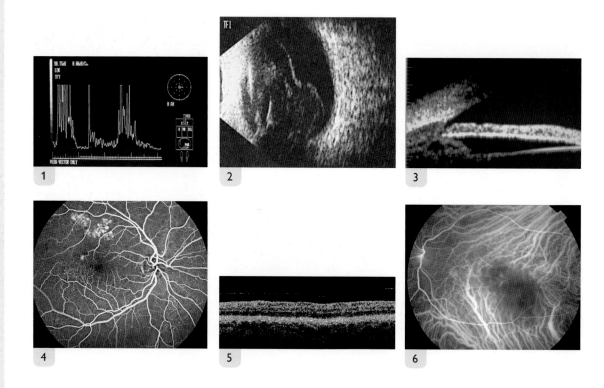

1

2

3

4

5

6

Answer on page 151

Q 92 What has caused these inferior forniceal conditions?

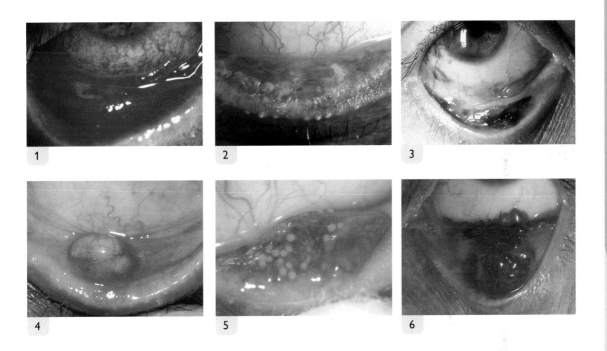

1   2   3

4   5   6

Answer on page 152

Q 93 What are these multiple signs?

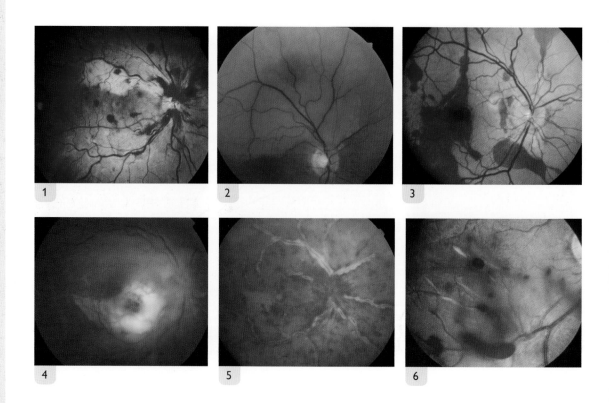

1

2

3

4

5

6

Answer on page 152

Q 94 What are these tests?

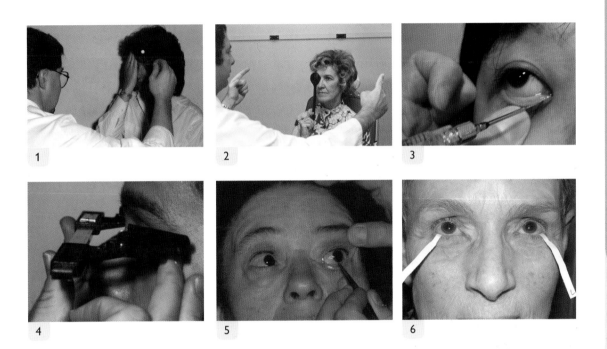

Answer on pages 152–153

Q 95 What are these subtle conditions?

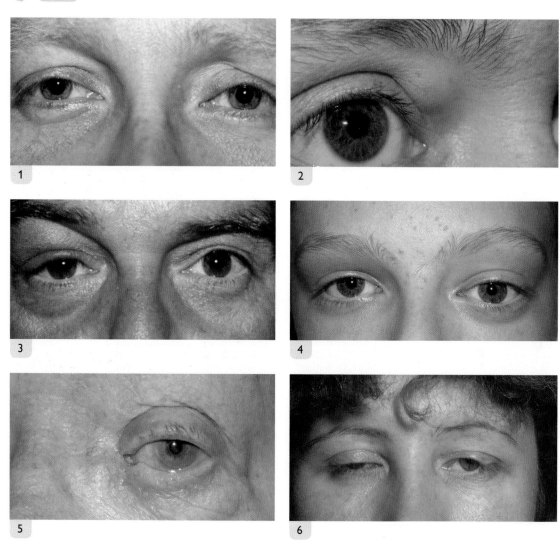

Answer on pages 153–154

Q 96   What are these ocular motility defects?

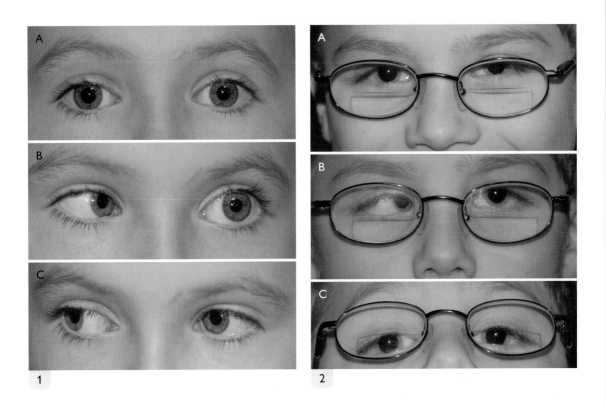

Answer on page 154

Q 97 Match the fundus (1–3) with the scan (A–C)

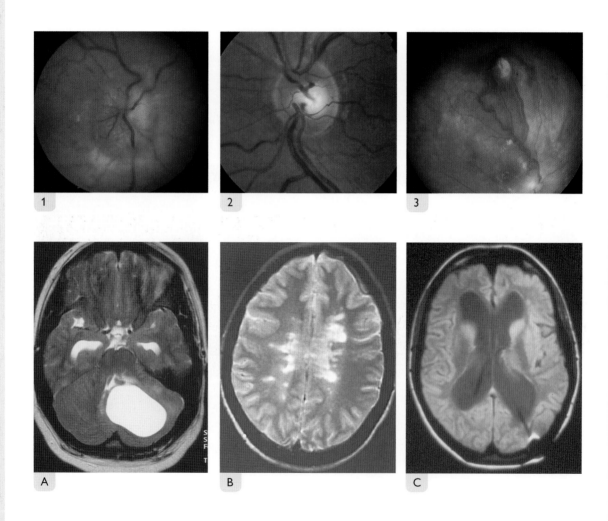

Answer on pages 154–155

Q **98** What has caused these atrophic iris lesions?

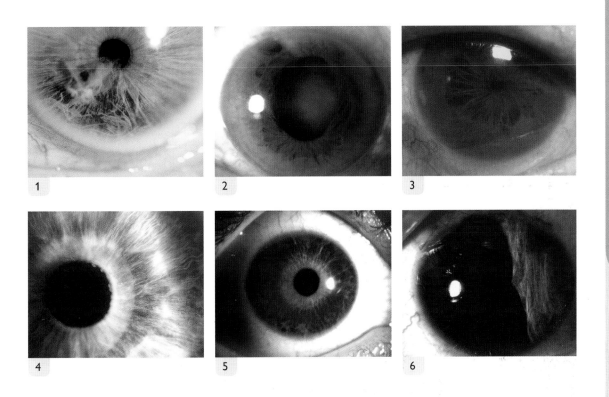

1

2

3

4

5

6

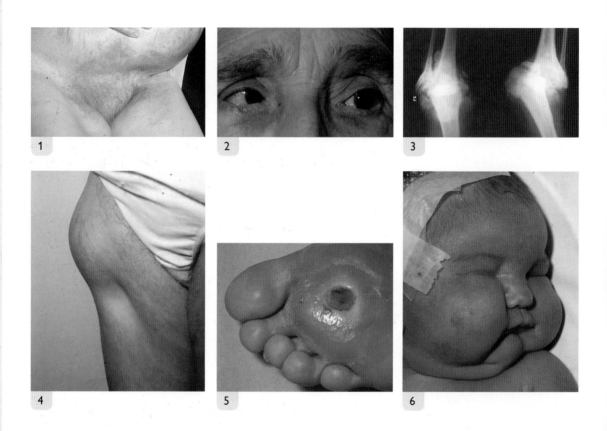

Q 99 What systemic disease has caused these problems?

1

2

3

4

5

6

Answer on page 155

Q 100 What do these angiograms show?

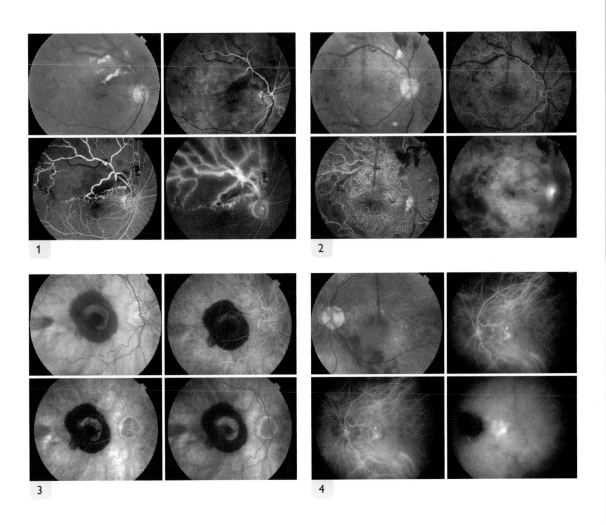

1

2

3

4

Answer on page 156

2 Answers

51 to 100

QUESTION 51

What are these malignancies?

1. Choroidal melanoma extends through the sclera by invading scleral channels and nerves. This carries a very poor prognosis as it indicates that the tumour is advanced and aggressive, and there is a risk of orbital spread.

2. Spreading sebaceous gland carcinoma is characterized by infiltration of the epidermis (pagetoid spread) that causes a diffuse thickening of the lid margin and may result in loss of lashes and be mistaken for 'chronic blepharitis'. It should be noted that chronic marginal blepharitis is always bilateral. Nodular sebaceous gland carcinoma may masquerade as 'recurrent chalazion'.

3. Metastatic carcinoma to iris is rare and may be characterized by multiple small pale nodules or a solitary, fast-growing mass. Anterior uveitis and occasionally spontaneous hyphaema may occur.

4. Small juxtapapillary choroidal melanoma should be distinguished from a choroidal naevus because it is more than 1 mm in thickness and 5 mm in diameter. Serial examinations by ultrasonography can be used to document growth.

5. Metastatic carcinoma to the choroid is characterized by often multiple, fast-growing, creamy-white placoid lesions. The most frequent primary sites are breast and bronchus. Less common primary sites are gastrointestinal tract, kidney, and skin melanoma.

6. Early intraretinal retinoblastoma is a small white plaque which may be detected on routine examination in a patient at risk or one with an established tumour in the fellow eye.

QUESTION 52

Match the eyelash disorders (1–3) with the aetiology (A–C)

1 and A

Acquired distichiasis (metaplastic lashes) is caused by metaplasia and dedifferentiation of the meibomian glands to become hair follicles which produce lashes (**1**). Unlike congenital distichiasis, the cilia tend to be non-pigmented and stunted, and cause ocular irritation. The most important cause is late stage cicatrizing conjunctivitis associated with chemical injury, ocular cicatricial pemphigoid, and **Stevens–Johnson syndrome**, which manifests an erythematous papular rash (**A**).

2 and C

Trichiasis is misdirection of lashes that arise from normal sites of origin (**2**). The condition may occur in isolation or as a result of scarring of the lid margin secondary to **herpes zoster ophthalmicus** (**C**) or severe chronic marginal blepharitis.

3 and B

Eyelash ptosis is a downward sagging of upper lashes (**3**). The condition may be idiopathic or associated with long-standing **facial palsy** (**B**), dermatochalasis, and floppy eyelid syndrome.

QUESTION 53

What are these items?

1. Plaque with seeds used for brachytherapy of intraocular tumours. The inner part of the plaque contains the radioactive source (ruthenium-106 or iodine-125) and the outer part is lined with a heavy metal such as gold or silver, to prevent radiation of nearby extraocular tissues.

2. Lester Jones tube insertion is indicated when there is either canalicular obstruction less than 8 mm from the puncta, or lacrimal pump failure.

3. Lacrimal stent tubes are occasionally used following revision surgery of failed dacryocystorhinostomy.

4. Schiotz tonometer relies on the principle of indentation tonometry in which a plunger with a pre-set weight indents the cornea. The amount of indentation is measured on a scale and the reading is converted into mmHg on a special table. The instrument is now seldom used because it is not as accurate as applanation tonometry.

QUESTION 54

What are the geographic connotations of these conditions?

1. Sands of Sahara (diffuse lamellar keratitis) is a complication of laser in-situ keratomileusis (LASEK) and is characterized by granular deposits at the flap interface.

2. Pyramidal cataract is a congenital conical anterior polar opacity that projects into the anterior chamber.

3. Sunset syndrome is a very rare complication that occurs months or years after cataract surgery in which the intraocular implant dislocates inferiorly into the vitreous. Rarely, it may be precipitated by laser capsulotomy.

4. Berlin oedema (commotio retinae) is caused by concussion of the sensory retina resulting in cloudy swelling which gives the involved area a grey appearance. The prognosis in mild cases is good with spontaneous resolution without sequelae within 6 weeks. Severe cases may lead to progressive pigmentary degeneration and macular hole formation.

5. Labrador keratopathy (spheroidal degeneration, climatic droplet keratopathy, and Bietti nodular dystrophy) is a bilateral condition which typically occurs in men whose working lives are spent outdoors. It is characterized by amber-coloured granules in the superficial stroma of the peripheral interpalpebral cornea that gradually increase in size and then coalesce.

6. North Carolina macular dystrophy is a very rare AD non-progressive condition. It was first described in families living in the mountains of North Carolina and subsequently in many unrelated families in other parts of the world. Grade 2 is characterized by deep, confluent macular deposits that may be occasionally complicated by choroidal neovascularization.

QUESTION 55

End-stage disease of which conditions?

1. Retinoblastoma with gross extraocular spread.

2. Thyrotoxicosis causing bilateral proptosis, exposure keratopathy, and panophthalmitis.

3. Congenital glaucoma causing gross buphthalmos, scleral thinning, and corneal scarring.

4. Chronic anterior uveitis causing phthisis bulbi and band keratopathy.

5. Cicatrizing conjunctivitis causing total symblepharon and corneal scarring.

6. Mooren ulcer causing total corneal destruction.

QUESTION 56

What treatment has been performed?

1. Tissue adhesive (cyanoacrylate) glue may be used to limit stromal ulceration and to seal small perforations. It is first applied onto a plastic patch, which is then applied to the cornea and a bandage contact lens is inserted.

2. Argon laser ablation may be used to treat scattered aberrant lashes. The initial settings are 50 μm,

0.2 sec and 1000 mW. The laser is fired at the root of the lash and a small crater formed. The spot size is increased to 200 μm and the crater deepened to reach the follicle. About a dozen applications are required and most patients are cured by one or two sessions.

3. Anterior subconjunctival injection of a long-acting corticosteroid such as triamcinolone acetonide (Kenalog) or a depot preparation such as methylprednisolone acetate (Depomedrone) may be used to control chronic anterior uveitis in cases resistant to topical administration or in non-compliant patients.

4. Small corneo-scleral patch graft may be required to seal peripheral corneal perforations where the use of glue is not appropriate.

5. Evisceration involves the removal of intraocular contents with preservation of the scleral shell and extraocular muscle attachments. A spherical orbital implant is also inserted. The procedure must be performed meticulously as leaving behind any uveal tissue can lead to sympathetic ophthalmitis.

6. Intrastromal corneal ring segment implantation into the peripheral cornea may be used to treat myopia and astigmatism. The procedure is relatively safe and has the advantage of being reversible and adjustable.

QUESTION 57

What has caused these superior tarsal lesions?

1. Atopic keratoconjunctivitis is a rare bilateral and symmetrical disease that typically develops in young men following a long history of severe atopic dermatitis. About 5% of patients have childhood vernal disease. Scarring and infiltration of the tarsal conjunctiva results in flattening of papillae, and a featureless appearance.

2. Ligneous conjunctivitis is a very rare disorder characterized by recurrent, often bilateral, firm, fibrin rich, woody-like pseudomembranous lesions that develop mainly on the tarsal conjunctiva. The lesions may be covered by a yellow-white thick mucoid discharge.

3. Spreading sebaceous gland carcinoma may occasionally diffusely infiltrate the conjunctival epithelium and may be mistaken for an inflammatory condition such as unilateral chronic blepharoconjunctivitis, superior limbic keratoconjunctivitis or cicatricial pemphigoid (masquerade syndrome).

4. Adenoviral conjunctivitis with pseudomembranes consisting of coagulated exudate adherent to the inflamed conjunctival epithelium that can be easily peeled off leaving the epithelium intact. True membranes infiltrate the superficial layers of the conjunctival epithelium so that attempted removal may be accompanied by tearing of the epithelium and bleeding. The distinction between a true membrane and a pseudomembrane is rarely clinically helpful as both can leave scarring following resolution.

5. Adrenochrome conjunctival deposits may occur from long-term use of topical adrenaline (epinephrine) for glaucoma. Because it is not as effective as other preparations such as beta-blockers and prostaglandin analogues it is now seldom used.

6. Superior limbic keratoconjunctivitis is an uncommon, usually bilateral, chronic disease characterized by papillary hypertrophy of the superior tarsal conjunctiva, hyperaemia of the superior bulbar conjunctiva, limbal papillary hypertrophy, and superior filamentary keratitis. It typically affects middle-aged women who have hyperthyroidism.

QUESTION 58

What is this systemic disease?

Lymphoma

Adnexal lymphoma may affect the **orbit** (**1**). Occasionally the tumour may be confined to the conjunctiva or lacrimal glands, sparing the orbit. **Conjunctival** lymphoma is characterized by a mobile, salmon-pink or flesh-coloured infiltrate in the fornices (**2**) or epibulbar surface. Primary intraocular lymphoma represents a subset of primary central nervous system lymphoma, which is a variant of extranodal non-Hodgkin lymphoma. **The lymphoma cells** are large, pleomorphic B lymphocytes with large multilobular nuclei, prominent nucleoli, and scanty cytoplasm (**3**). The tumour arises from within the **brain** (**4**), spinal cord, and leptomeninges. Intraocular involvement is characterized by multifocal, large, yellowish, **solid sub-RPE infiltrates** (**5**). **Vitritis** is common and may impede visualization of the fundus (**6**).

QUESTION 59

What types of ptosis are shown?

1. Simple congenital ptosis may be unilateral or bilateral and of variable severity. It is associated with a poorly developed or absent upper lid crease, and limited levator function.

2. Mechanical ptosis may be caused by tumours, oedema, scarring, anterior orbital lesions, and dermatochalasis.

3. Neurogenic ptosis due to Horner syndrome (oculosympathetic palsy) is characterized by mild ptosis, ipsilateral miosis, slight elevation of the inferior eyelid and normal pupillary reactions to light and near. Reduced ipsilateral sweating may be present, if the lesion is below the superior cervical ganglion.

4. Aponeurotic ptosis is caused by dehiscence, disinsertion or stretching of the levator aponeurosis which restricts transmission of force from a normal levator muscle to the upper lid. Involutional aponeurotic ptosis is characterized by usually bilateral ptosis with a high upper lid crease and good levator function. In severe cases the upper lid crease may be absent, the eyelid above the tarsal plate very thin, and the upper sulcus deep.

5. Neurogenic ptosis due to third nerve palsy is caused by innervational levator weakness. Ptosis is usually severe and is associated with ophthalmoplegia. Mydriasis is also present if the cause of the third nerve palsy is due to a 'surgical lesion' such as an aneurysm, trauma or uncal herniation.

6. Myogenic ptosis due to myasthenia gravis is insidious, bilateral, and frequently asymmetrical. It is worse on prolonged upgaze due to fatigue, and may be associated with diplopia, which is often vertical.

QUESTION 60

What are these orthoptic instruments?

1. The Titmus test consists of a three-dimensional Polaroid vectograph consisting of two plates in the form of a booklet which is viewed through Polaroid spectacles. On the right is a large fly, and on the left is a series of circles and animals. The test is performed at a distance of 40 cm and is used to test stereopsis.

2. The Lees screen consists of two opalescent glass screens at right-angles to each other, bisected by a two-sided plane mirror which dissociates the two eyes. Each screen has a tangent pattern marked onto the back surface which is revealed only when the screen is illuminated. It is used in the investigation of diplopia.

3. Bagolini striated glasses are used to detect binocular single vision, anomalous retinal correspondence, and suppression. Each lens has fine striations which convert a point source of light into a line.

4. Maddox rod consists of a series of fused cylindrical red glass rods which convert the appearance of a white spot of light into a red streak. The optical properties of the rods cause the streak of light to be at an angle of 90° with the long axis of the rods; when the glass rods are held horizontally, the streak will be vertical and vice versa.

5. The synoptophore consists of two cylindrical tubes with a mirrored right-angled bend and a +6.50 D lens in each eyepiece. This optically sets the testing distance as equivalent to about 6 metres. Pictures are inserted in a slide carrier situated at the outer end of each tube. The two tubes are supported on columns which enable the pictures to be moved in relation to each other, and any adjustments are indicated on a scale. The synoptophore can measure horizontal, vertical, and torsional misalignments and can be used in the investigation of sensory abnormalities.

6. The RAF rule is used to measure the near point of convergence which is the nearest point on which the eyes can maintain binocular fixation. It can also measure the near point of accommodation which is the nearest point on which the eyes can maintain clear focus.

QUESTION 61

Match the fundus (1–3) with the scan (A–C)

1 and C

Terson syndrome refers to the combination of intraocular haemorrhage and subarachnoid haemorrhage secondary to aneurysmal rupture, most commonly arising from the circle of Willis. The haemorrhage is frequently bilateral, and intraretinal and/or subhyaloid (**1**), although occasionally subhyaloid blood may break into the vitreous. **CT** in patients with subarachnoid haemorrhages shows intraventricular blood (**C**).

2 and B

Optic nerve sheath meningiomas arise from meningothelial cells of the arachnoid villi surrounding the intraorbital or, less commonly, the intracanalicular portion of the optic nerve. The classical triad is visual loss, optic atrophy and opticociliary shunt vessels (**2**). However, the simultaneous occurrence of all three signs in one individual is uncommon. Coronal **CT** shows thickening and calcification of the right optic nerve (**B**).

3 and A

Pituitary adenomas may compress the optic nerves and give rise to optic atrophy (**3**), especially if the chiasm is located more posteriorly over the dorsum sellae (postfixed chiasm). T1-weighted gadolinium enhanced **MR** sagittal view shows a large pituitary adenoma (**A**).

QUESTION 62

What are these signs?

1. Sentinel sign describes dilated episcleral blood vessels in the same quadrant as a ciliary body melanoma.

2. Eclipse sign occurs in eyes with shallow anterior chambers and is demonstrated by shining a light from the temporal side. Because of the convexity of the iris-lens diaphragm, the nasal iris manifests a crescentic shadow.

3. Bayoneting occurs in a glaucomatous disc and is characterized by double angulation of a blood vessel as it dives sharply backwards and then turns along the steep wall of the excavation before angling again onto the floor of the disc.

4. 'T' sign demonstrates posterior scleritis. Ultrasonography shows fluid in Tenon space in which the T is formed by the optic nerve on its side and the cross bar by the gap containing fluid.

5. Dermatographism demonstrates a sensitive skin in patients with Behçet disease in which erythematous lines appear following stroking of the skin.

6. Tobacco dust is characterized by the presence of pigment cells in the anterior vitreous gel. It strongly correlates with the presence of a retinal tear even in the absence of retinal detachment.

QUESTION 63

What are these complications of intraocular lens implantation?

1. Iris bombé due to pupil block occurs following implantation of an anterior chamber IOL when a peripheral iridotomy has not been performed or is inadequate.

2. Decentration of a posterior chamber IOL may occur if one haptic is inserted into the sulcus and the other into the capsular bag, or rarely the angle.

3. Partial prolapse into the anterior chamber of one haptic of an anterior chamber IOL may occur if the pupil is not well miosed following completion of surgery.

4. Dislocation into the anterior chamber of a posterior chamber IOL may result in endothelial damage and corneal oedema.

5. Dislocation into the vitreous of a posterior chamber IOL is an extremely rare but very serious complication that reflects inappropriate implantation. Complications include uveitis, vitreous haemorrhage, retinal detachment, and cystoid macular oedema.

6. Opacification of an IOL is extremely rare.

QUESTION 64

What are these subtle conditions?

1. Fine macular drusen are innocuous.

2. Resolving cytomegalovirus retinitis with residual granularity at the inferior posterior pole. Initially 95% of cases respond to treatment but all relapse within 2 weeks when therapy is discontinued. There is a 50% relapse rate within 6 months in patients on maintenance therapy.

3. Toxoplasma retinitis with a small focus just below the superior vascular arcade. The diagnosis

toxoplasma retinitis is based on a compatible fundus lesion and positive serology for toxoplasma antibodies. Any antibody titre is significant and in recurrent ocular toxoplasmosis, no correlation exists between the titre and the activity of retinitis.

4. Angioid streaks with mottled 'peau d'orange' (orange skin) pigmentation in the temporal fundus. Approximately 50% of patients with angioid streaks have one of the following conditions: pseudoxanthoma elasticum (most common), Ehlers–Danlos syndrome type 6 (ocular sclerotic), Paget disease, and haemoglobinopathies.

5. Cavernous retinal haemangioma is characterized by a cluster of small aneurysms resembling a bunch of grapes. It is a rare, congenital, hamartoma which is usually innocuous but can occasionally give rise to vitreous haemorrhage.

6. Shallow supero-temporal retinal detachment in which the area of detachment has a slightly opaque and corrugated appearance as a result of intraretinal oedema. There is loss of the underlying choroidal pattern and retinal blood vessels appear darker than in flat retina, so that the colour contrast between veins and arteries is less apparent.

QUESTION 65

What treatment has been performed?

1. Laser photocoagulation of a retinal break may be considered in cases that carry a significant risk of subsequent retinal detachment. This includes most retinal tears, particularly if large and symptomatic.

2. Intravitreal heavy liquid injection combined with vitrectomy has greatly improved the success rate of treatment of retinal detachment due to giant retinal tears.

3. Trans-scleral choroidectomy for choroidal melanoma is a difficult procedure that is not widely performed. It may be considered for carefully selected cases that are too thick for radiotherapy and usually less than 16 mm in diameter.

4. YAG laser coagulation of a large subhyaloid haemorrhage is rarely performed as most cases are unilateral and absorb spontaneously. Laser therapy may be considered in long-standing cases in patients with poor vision in the fellow eye.

5. Scleral buckling for retinal detachment is a surgical procedure in which material sutured onto the sclera (explant) creates an inward indentation (buckle). Its purposes are to close retinal breaks by apposing the RPE to the sensory retina, and to reduce dynamic vitreoretinal traction at sites of local vitreoretinal adhesion. The explant may be placed radially, circumferentially or it may encircle the globe.

6. Slow-release intravitreal steroid implants are currently being developed. They contain an insoluble steroid (fluocinolone acetonide) that is continuously released for 3 years and may obviate the long-term use of systemic steroids.

QUESTION 66

Who invented?

1. Trabeculectomy was invented in 1968 by John Cairns, a British ophthalmologist working in Cambridge. The procedure was subsequently modified by his colleague Peter Watson. Trabeculectomy lowers intraocular pressure by the creation of a fistula that allows aqueous outflow from the anterior chamber to sub-Tenon space. The fistula is protected or 'guarded' by a superficial scleral flap.

2. Goniotomy was invented by Otto Barkan (1857–1958), an American ophthalmologist. In 1936 he presented the results of a procedure in which he incised through the trabecular meshwork into Schlemm canal. Goniotomy is still widely used to treat congenital glaucoma and has a high success rate provided the condition is not advanced and there is good visualization of the angle.

3. Brachytherapy for choroidal melanoma was invented in 1948 by Hyla 'Henry' Stallard (1901–1973), a British ophthalmologist working at St. Bartholomew's Hospital in London. Stallard was a bronze medallist in the 1500 metres in the 1924 Olympic Games. Brachytherapy involves the use of radioactive plaques which are secured onto the sclera over the tumour.

4. Hand-held applanation tonometry was invented by Terry Perkins, a British ophthalmologist. It is particularly useful in bed-bound or anaesthetized patients.

5. Indirect ophthalmoscopy was invented by Charles Schepens (1912–2006), a Belgian ophthalmologist working in the USA, who made many other important contributions in the field of retinal detachment.

6. Fundus fluorescein angiography was first performed successfully on a human in 1961 by American scientists H Novotny and D Alvis.

QUESTION 67

Match the conjunctival lesion (1–3) with the histology (A–C)

1 and B

Conjunctival follicles are multiple, discrete, yellowish, slightly elevated lesions, most prominent in the fornices (**1**). Their size is related to severity and duration of disease. Vessels normally pass over the surface of the follicle and as it increases in size, they are displaced peripherally. **Histology** shows a subepithelial germinal centre with immature lymphocytes centrally and mature cells peripherally (**B**). Causes include: viral conjunctivitis, chlamydial conjunctivitis, Parinaud oculoglandular syndrome, and hypersensitivity to topical medications.

2 and C

Nodular conjunctival squamous cell carcinoma is a fleshy, pink papillomatous mass with feeder vessels often at the limbus but may be anywhere (**2**). Metastasis can rarely occur to regional lymph nodes and systemically. **Histology** shows downward proliferation of irregular, dysplastic, squamous epithelium with infiltration of subepithelial tissue (**C**).

3 and A

Conjunctival papillae can only develop in the palpebral conjunctiva and the limbal bulbar conjunctiva where it is attached to the deeper fibrous layer. Micropapillae form a mosaic-like pattern of elevated red dots as a result of the central vascular channel. Macropapillae (<1 mm) (**3**) and giant papillae (>1 mm) develop with prolonged inflammation. **Histology** shows folds of hyperplastic conjunctival epithelium with a fibrovascular core and subepithelial stromal infiltration with inflammatory cells (**A**). Causes include: chronic blepharitis, allergic conjunctivitis, bacterial conjunctivitis, contact lens wear, superior limbic keratoconjunctivitis, and floppy eyelid syndrome.

QUESTION 68

Match the keratitis (1–3) with the pathogen (A–C)

1 and A

Acanthamoeba keratitis is most frequently associated with contact lens wear, especially if tap water is use for cleaning. A ring infiltrate is characteristic in established disease (**1**). **Staining** using periodic acid–Schiff or calcofluor white, a fluorescent dye with an affinity for amoebic cysts and fungi, may be used for identification (**A**). It should be noted that pain may be severe and disproportionate to the clinical signs.

2 and C

Dendritic herpes simplex keratitis is characterized by ulceration with linear branches that stains with fluorescein (**2**). Transmission **electron microscopy** may be used to demonstrate the virus (**C**).

3 and B

Gonococcal keratitis occurs when conjunctivitis is not appropriately treated. Initially corneal ulceration is peripheral and frequently superior (**3**). **Gram staining** shows Gram-negative kidney-shaped diplococci (**B**).

QUESTION 69

What are these neuroimaging techniques?

1. Computed tomography (CT) uses x-ray beams to obtain tissue density values from which detailed cross-sectional images are formed by a computer. Tissue density is represented by a grey scale, white being maximum density (e.g. bone) and black being minimum density (e.g. air). Iodinated contrast material improves sensitivity and specificity but is not indicated in the assessment of acute haemorrhage, bony injury or localization of foreign bodies because it may mask visualization of these high density structures.

2. Magnetic resonance imaging (MR) depends on the rearrangement of hydrogen nuclei (protons – positively charged) when a tissue is exposed to a short electromagnetic pulse. When the pulse subsides, the nuclei return to their normal position re-radiating some of the energy they have absorbed. Sensitive receivers pick up this electromagnetic echo. Weighting refers to two methods of measuring the relaxation times of the excited protons after the magnetic field has been switched off. T1-weighted images are best for normal anatomy. Hypointense (dark) structures include CSF and vitreous. Hyperintense (bright) structures include fat, blood, and contrast agents. T2-weighted images are useful for viewing pathological changes because water is hyperintense. It should be noted that bone and calcification are poorly visualized on MR.

3. Magnetic resonance angiography (MRA) is a non-invasive method of imaging the intra- and extracranial carotids and vertebrobasilar circulations to demonstrate stenosis, dissection, occlusion, arteriovenous malformations, and aneurysms provided they are not too small.

4. Computed tomography venography may be useful when MRA is contraindicated or there are difficulties in distinguishing slow flow from thrombus on MRA. However it is not as sensitive as MRA in detecting associated parenchymal changes and this usually limits its use to equivocal cases.

5. Computed tomography angiography (CTA) is emerging as the method of choice in the investigation of intracranial aneurysms. It enables acquisition of extremely thin slice images of the brain following intravenous contrast. Images of the vessels can be reconstructed in three dimensions and viewed in any direction on a workstation. The investigation is safe and quick and without the 1% risk of stroke that is carried with conventional catheter angiography.

6. Conventional intra-arterial catheter angiography involves the passage of a catheter via the femoral artery into the internal carotid and vertebral arteries in the neck under fluoroscopic guidance. Following contrast injection images are taken in rapid succession. Digital subtraction results in images of the contrast-filled vessels without any background structure such as bone. Until recently, this technique was the first line investigation in the diagnosis of intracranial aneurysms. This remains true in some centres where CTA is a relatively new technique and in cases where CTA is equivocal or negative.

QUESTION 70

Match the lashes (1–3) with the skin (A–C)

I and B

Congenital distichiasis is a partial or complete second row of lashes emerging at or slightly behind the meibomian gland orifices. The aberrant lashes tend to be thinner and shorter than normal cilia and are often directed posteriorly (**1**). The condition is frequently inherited in an AD manner and associated with **lymphoedema** of the legs (**B**) (lymphoedema-distichiasis syndrome).

2 and C

Poliosis is a premature localized whitening of hair, which may involve the lashes (**2**) and eyebrows. Some patients also exhibit **vitiligo** which consists of sharply defined white macules which are often symmetrical (**C**). Systemic associations of poliosis include: Vogt–Koyanagi–Harada syndrome, Waardenburg syndrome, Marfan syndrome, and tuberous sclerosis.

3 and A

Madarosis is a decrease in the number of lashes (**3**) that may be due to local causes or part of a **generalized alopecia** (**A**). Systemic causes of madarosis include: myxoedema, systemic lupus erythematosus, acquired syphilis, and lepromatous leprosy.

QUESTION 71

Toxoplasmosis or toxocariasis?

1. Toxocaral granuloma at the posterior pole is associated with fibrosis, distortion of vasculature, and mild temporal traction of the optic nerve head. It presents between the ages of 6 and 14 years with visual loss. Ocular toxocariasis is always unilateral and occurs in an otherwise healthy child.

2. Toxoplasmosis resulting in hydrocephalus and left anophthalmos. Severity of fetal involvement is dependent on the duration of gestation at the time of maternal infestation. Involvement during early pregnancy may result in stillbirth, whereas if it occurs during late pregnancy it may cause CNS and visceral disease.

3. Toxocaral granuloma on the optic disc is uncommon and may give rise to diagnostic difficulties.

4. Toxoplasma retinitis with severe vitritis resulting in a 'headlight in the fog' appearance.

5. Toxocara causing a vitreoretinal band extending from the posterior pole to the periphery. Ultrasonography is useful in establishing a diagnosis in eyes with hazy media and excluding other causes of leukocoria, notably retinoblastoma.

6. Toxoplasma resulting in an atrophic scar at the macula present at birth is caused by intrauterine infection towards the end of the second trimester.

QUESTION 72

What is the underlying causes of the hard exudates?

1. Coats disease is an idiopathic, non-hereditary, retinal telangiectasis characterized by intraretinal and subretinal exudation, and frequently exudative retinal detachment. About 75% of patients are males and the vast majority have uniocular involvement.

2. Old branch retinal vein occlusion is characterized by venous sheathing, collaterals, residual retinal haemorrhages, and hard exudates.

3. Juxtapapillary haemangioblastoma is a rare sight-threatening tumour that is very strongly associated with von Hippel–Lindau disease, although it may occasionally occur in isolation. It is characterized by a well-defined round orange-red mass that may be surrounded by hard exudates. A peripheral tumour may cause exudation at the macula.

4. End-stage wet age-related macular degeneration may be associated with massive subretinal exudation as a result of chronic leakage from choroidal neovascularization.

5. Retinal artery macroaneurysm is a localized dilatation of a retinal arteriole which usually occurs in the first three orders of the arterial tree. Associated retinal haemorrhage is present in 50% of cases. Chronic leakage resulting in retinal oedema with accumulation of hard exudates at the fovea is common and may result in permanent loss of central vision.

6. Background diabetic retinopathy is characterized by hard exudates arranged in rings that may be complete or incomplete, microaneurysms, and dot and blot haemorrhages.

QUESTION 73

What are these instruments?

1. Goniotomy needle and infusion syringe used to treat primary congenital glaucoma. Goniotomy is performed provided there is sufficient corneal clarity and the angle can be visualized. The procedure involves making a horizontal incision at the midpoint of the superficial layers of the trabecular meshwork. Although goniotomy may need to be repeated, the eventual success rate is about 85%.

2. Ultrasonic biomicroscope utilizes high frequency ultrasound at 30–50 MHz that provides high-definition imaging of the anterior segment but only to a depth of 5 mm. It is of particular value in the evaluation of eyes with congenital corneal opacification.

3. Mini vitrector is used to obtain vitreous samples for bacteriology in eyes with endophthalmitis.

4. Tono-Pen is a hand-held, self-contained, battery powered, portable, contact tonometer. It correlates well with Goldmann tonometry although it slightly overestimates a low IOP and underestimates a high IOP. Its main advantage is the ability to measure IOP in eyes with distorted or oedematous corneas, as well as through a bandage contact lens.

5. Non-contact tonometer is based on the principle of applanation but, instead of using a prism, the central part of the cornea is flattened by a jet of air. The time required to sufficiently flatten the cornea relates directly to the level of IOP. The instrument is easy to use and does not require topical anaesthesia. It is therefore particularly useful for screening by non-ophthalmologists. Its main disadvantage is that it is accurate only within the low-to-middle range.

6. Cryoprobe for ablating lashes is very effective in eliminating many troublesome lashes as in severe trichiasis and distichiasis. A double freeze-thaw cycle at −20°C is applied. Potential complications include skin necrosis, depigmentation in dark-skinned individuals, damage to meibomian glands (which may adversely affect the precorneal tear film), and shallow notching of the lid margin.

QUESTION 74

What are these subtle lesions?

1. Conjunctival naevus is a benign, usually unilateral, lesion. Presentation is during the first two decades of life with solitary, flat or slightly elevated, pigmented intraepithelial bulbar lesion most frequently in the juxtalimbal area. The extent of pigmentation is variable and some may be virtually non-pigmented.

2. Lisch nodules are, small, bilateral, iris naevi found after the age of 16 years in virtually all patients with neurofibromatosis-1.

3. Increased scleral translucency may follow resolution of anterior non-necrotizing scleritis. As the oedema resolves the affected areas often take on a slight grey/blue appearance because of increased scleral translucency due to rearrangement of scleral fibres rather than a decrease in scleral thickness.

4. Conjunctivochalasis is characterized by a fold of redundant conjunctiva interposed between the globe and lower eyelid that protrudes over the lid margin. The inferior cornea stains with Rose Bengal. Conjunctivochalasis is probably a normal ageing change that may be exacerbated by posterior lid margin disease. Mechanical stress on the conjunctiva precipitated by dry eye is a potential mechanism.

5. Dellen is an innocuous localized, saucer-like thinning of the peripheral cornea resulting from dehydration of the stroma and compaction of its lamellae. It is caused by localized tear film instability that may be idiopathic or secondary to raised limbal lesions.

6. Detachment of Descemet membrane is a rare complication of cataract surgery. Unless repaired it may lead to endothelial decompensation and corneal oedema.

QUESTION 75

Match the mouth (1–3) with the eye (A–C)

1 and B

Marfan syndrome is a widespread disorder of connective tissue associated with mutation of the fibrillin gene on chromosome 15q. Inheritance is AD with variable expressivity. A narrow high-arched (gothic) palate is characteristic (**1**). Other features include: tall and thin stature, disproportionately long limbs compared with the trunk (arm span > height) and long spider-like fingers and toes (arachnodactyly). Ectopia lentis which is bilateral, symmetrical, and most frequently supero-temporal (**B**) is present in 80% of cases.

2 and A

Behçet syndrome is an idiopathic, multisystem disease characterized by recurrent episodes of oro-genital ulceration, and vasculitis which may involve small, medium, and large veins and arteries. Oral ulceration is characterized by recurrent painful aphthous lesions (**2**). Acute recurrent anterior uveitis which may be simultaneously bilateral is common. It is frequently associated with a transient mobile hypopyon in a relatively white eye (**A**). It is often a mild manifestation when compared to posterior segment involvement and usually responds well to topical steroids.

3 and C

Mucous membrane pemphigoid is an autoimmune mucocutaneous blistering disease that may affect the mouth, nose, pharynx, trachea, genitalia, and anus. The condition affects women more commonly than men (2:1) with a peak age of onset after 70 years of age. Mucosal subepidermal blisters, most frequently oral (**3**), rupture within a day or two leaving erosions and ulcers that heal without significant scarring. Conjunctival disease (ocular cicatricial pemphigoid) is seen in 75% of cases with oral involvement but only in 25% of those with skin lesions. It is characterized by chronic conjunctivitis with subconjunctival fibrosis resulting in forniceal shortening and symblepharon formation (**C**).

QUESTION 76

Match the eye (1–3) with the treatment (A–C)

1 and B

Band keratopathy is a common condition characterized by the deposition of calcium salts in Bowman layer, epithelial basement membrane, and anterior stroma. It is characterized by peripheral interpalpebral calcification with clear cornea separating the sharp peripheral margins of the band from the limbus. This gradually spreads centrally to form a band-like chalky plaque containing transparent small holes and occasionally clefts (**1**). Treatment is indicated if vision is threatened or if the eye is uncomfortable. **Chelation** is simple and effective for relatively mild cases. First the corneal epithelium is removed and then a solution of ethylenediamine-tetra-acetic acid (EDTA) is applied with a cotton bud (**B**) until all calcium has been removed. Important causes of band keratopathy are chronic anterior uveitis (particularly in children), phthisis bulbi, and age-related.

2 and A

Intermediate uveitis is an insidious, chronic, relapsing disease in which the vitreous is the major site of the inflammation. The condition may be idiopathic or associated with a systemic disease. Pars planitis is a subset of idiopathic intermediate uveitis in which there is snowbanking (**2**) or snowball formation. Cystoid macular oedema occurs in 30% of cases and is the most common reason to initiate therapy which initially involves posterior sub-Tenon **injections of triamcinolone** (**A**). Systemic associations of intermediate uveitis include multiple sclerosis, sarcoidosis, and Lyme disease.

3 and C

Keratoconjunctivitis sicca describes a dry eye due to aqueous tear deficiency. Rose Bengal is a vital dye that has an affinity for dead and devitalized epithelial cells that have an abnormal mucous layer. Epithelial filaments and mucous plaques stain well with Rose Bengal, as does the dry interpalpebral conjunctiva (**3**). **Punctal occlusion** (**C**) reduces drainage and thereby preserves natural tears and prolongs the effect of artificial tears. It is of greatest value in patients with moderate to severe dryness who have not responded to topical treatment.

QUESTION 77

What has caused these iris transillumination defects?

1. Progressive iris atrophy has resulted in full-thickness iris defects.

2. Sectoral iris atrophy due to herpes zoster or **herpes simplex iritis** is caused by ischaemia due to occlusive vasculitis.

3. Diabetic iridopathy is characterized by spotty defects as a result of atrophy of the posterior pigment layer.

4. Circumferential iris atrophy in Fuchs uveitis syndrome. Advanced stromal atrophy makes the affected iris appear dull with loss of detail giving rise to a washed-out appearance, particularly in the pupillary zone. Posterior pigment layer iris atrophy is best detected by retroillumination.

5. Spoke-like iris atrophy in pigment dispersion syndrome which is caused by the liberation of pigment granules from the iris pigment epithelium and their deposition throughout the anterior segment. Pigment epithelial atrophy due to shedding of pigment from the mid-periphery gives rise to characteristic radial slit-like defects.

6. Diffuse iris atrophy in albinism. Albinism is a genetically determined, heterogeneous group of disorders of melanin synthesis in which either the eyes alone (ocular albinism) or the eyes, skin, and hair (oculocutaneous albinism) may be affected. The latter may be either tyrosinase-positive or tyrosinase-negative. Iris translucency is variable and gives rise to a 'pink eye' appearance. It is most severe in tyrosinase-negative patients.

QUESTION 78

What have these conditions in common?

They are associated with night blindness (nyctalopia)

1. Xerophthalmia is caused by vitamin A deficiency. It is responsible for up to 100,000 new cases of blindness worldwide each year and is the leading cause of childhood blindness. Symptoms are nyctalopia and ocular irritation due to dryness. Bitot spots are triangular patches of foamy keratinized epithelium in the interpalpebral zone (**1**) thought to be caused by infection with *Corynebacterium xerosis*. Retinopathy characterized by yellowish peripheral dots may occur in advanced cases and is associated with decreased ERG amplitude.

2. Oguchi disease is an AR condition in which the fundus has an unusual golden-yellow colour (**A**) in the light-adapted state which becomes normal after prolonged dark adaptation (Mizuo phenomenon – **B**).

3. Melanoma-associated retinopathy is a rare paraneoplastic syndrome associated with cutaneous melanoma (**3**). It presents with nyctalopia and shimmering or flickering lights followed by sudden loss of central vision. The fundus appears normal initially, but optic disc pallor, retinal vascular attenuation, and vitreous cells can develop subsequently. A 'negative ERG' pattern is characteristic and is similar to that seen in congenital stationary night blindness.

4. Fundus albipunctatus is an AR condition characterized by congenital stationary nyctalopia. The fundus shows a multitude of tiny yellow-white spots at the posterior pole, sparing the fovea, and extending to the periphery (**4**). The retinal blood vessels, optic disc, peripheral fields, and visual acuity remain normal. The ERG and EOG may be abnormal when tested routinely but revert to normal on prolonged dark adaptation.

5. Retinitis pigmentosa defines a clinically and genetically diverse group of diffuse retinal dystrophies initially predominantly affecting the rod photoreceptor cells with subsequent degeneration of cones. Presentation is with nyctalopia, often during the third decade, but may be sooner depending on the pedigree. The fundus shows arteriolar narrowing and perivascular 'bone-spicule' pigmentary changes (**5**).

6. Panretinal photocoagulation is performed for proliferative diabetic retinopathy. In severe cases a large area of the peripheral fundus has to be ablated to ensure regression of neovascularization. Patients who have had bilateral aggressive treatment (**6**) may complain of mild nyctalopia as well as restriction of visual fields.

QUESTION 79

What are these causes of leukocoria?

1. Coats disease is an idiopathic, non-hereditary, retinal telangiectasis characterized by intraretinal and subretinal exudation, and frequently exudative retinal detachment (**B**). Presentation is most frequently in the first decade of life (average 5 years) with unilateral leukocoria (**A**), visual loss or strabismus. Occasionally the condition may present in later childhood and rarely in adult life.

2. Retinoblastoma (**B**) typically presents within the first year of life in bilateral cases and around two years of age if the tumour is unilateral. About 60% of patients present with leukocoria (**A**). Although the parent's description is usually very accurate not all general practitioners are aware of the importance of this sign so that referral to an ophthalmologist may be delayed.

3. Chronic toxocaral endophthalmitis presents between the ages of 2 and 9 years with leukocoria (**A**), strabismus or unilateral visual loss. Associated anterior uveitis may result in the formation of posterior synechiae and an irregular pupil. The peripheral retina and pars plana may be covered by a dense grayish-white exudate, similar to the 'snowbanking' seen in pars planitis (**B**). Prognosis in most cases is very poor and some eyes eventually require enucleation.

QUESTION 80

What treatment is being performed?

1. Amniotic membrane transplantation utilizes the inner layer of the placenta to promote corneal epithelial healing and reduce ocular surface inflammation. It can be used to treat a variety of serious ocular surface disorders such as, persistent corneal epithelial defects, chemical injuries, neurotrophic ulceration, and ocular cicatricial pemphigoid.

2. Coil occlusion of an intracranial aneurysm involves the insertion of soft metallic coils within the lumen of the aneurysm thereby excluding the aneurysmal sac from the intracranial circulation while preserving the parent artery.

3. Lensectomy for persistent anterior fetal vasculature may be successful in selected mild cases in salvaging some vision. Excision of the lens and retrolental tissue clears the visual axis, improves cosmesis, and prevents angle-closure caused by shallowing of the anterior chamber.

4. Orbitotomy is performed for excision of tumours, decompression where increased intraorbital pressure threatens optic nerve function, and repair of orbital fractures. The surgical approaches may be anterior, lateral, medial, or superior, depending on the location of the lesion and the required exposure.

5. Argon laser suture lysis should be considered 7–14 days following trabeculectomy to promote drainage in eyes with high intraocular pressures, flat blebs, and deep anterior chambers. Lysis is performed through a Hoskins lens or a Zeiss four-mirror lens.

6. Retinal membrane peeling is performed, in conjunction with pars plana vitrectomy, to remove epiretinal membranes in eyes with proliferative vitreoretinopathy, tractional retinal detachments, and macular pucker. The two main techniques in removing fibrovascular membranes in diabetic tractional detachments are delamination and segmentation.

QUESTION 81

Which ophthalmologists described these?

1. Henning Ronne (1878–1947), a Danish ophthalmologist, described the **nasal step** glaucomatous defect, which represents a difference in sensitivity above and below the horizontal midline in the nasal field. It is a common finding usually associated with other visual field defects.

2. Marc Amsler (1891–1968), a Swiss ophthalmologist, devised the Amsler **grid** which is used to evaluate 20° of the visual field mainly in screening for macular disease.

3. Jannik Bjerrum (1851–1920), a Danish ophthalmologist, described a characteristic glaucomatous nerve fibre bundle **visual field defect** that extends from the blind spot, sweeps around the macula, and ends in a straight line on the nasal side corresponding to the temporal raphe.

4. Hans Goldmann (1899–1991), a Swiss ophthalmologist, described an indirect **goniolens** with a contact surface diameter of approximately 12 mm. It is relatively easy to master and affords an excellent view of the angle and peripheral retina. The original Goldmann lens has three mirrors. Modifications with one mirror and two mirrors with an antireflective coating have been designed for laser trabeculoplasty, enabling simultaneous visualization of a wider circumference of the angle.

5. D. Jackson Coleman, an American ophthalmologist, together with Frederic Lizzi, created the first commercially available **B-scan ultrasound** equipment.

6. Leonhard Koeppe (1884–1969), a German ophthalmologist, described a dome-shaped direct diagnostic **goniolens** which comes in several sizes. It provides a panoramic view of the angle and is particularly useful for simultaneous comparison of one portion of the angle with another. Moreover, with the patient in the supine position the anterior chamber may become slightly deeper and the angle easier to identify.

QUESTION 82

Benign or malignant eyelid lesions?

1. Benign – capillary haemangioma is the most common tumour of the orbit and periorbital area in childhood. Histology shows proliferation of very small diameter vascular channels within the dermis lined by bland endothelium.

2. Malignant – squamous cell carcinoma is much less common but more aggressive than basal cell carcinoma. The tumour may arise *de novo* or from pre-existing actinic keratosis. Histology shows acanthotic squamous epithelium and islands of dysplastic squamous epithelium within the dermis.

3. Benign – chalazion is a chronic, sterile, granulomatous inflammatory lesion caused by retained sebaceous secretion leaking from the meibomian glands or other sebaceous glands into adjacent stroma. Histology shows a lipogranulomatous inflammatory reaction containing epithelioid and multinucleated giant cells intermixed with lymphocytes and plasma cells. The well-demarcated empty space is from where fat was dissolved out during processing.

4. Benign – intradermal naevus typically presents in old age as a papillomatous lesion with little if any pigmentation. Histology shows irregular clusters of bland darkly staining naevus cells.

5. Malignant – melanoma is rare. The two main types are superficial spreading and nodular. Histology shows a very extensive population of pigment-laden large atypical melanocytes within the dermis.

6. Benign – plexiform neurofibroma typically affects the upper eyelids of patients with neurofibromatosis-1. Histology shows proliferation of Schwann cells, fibroblasts and nerve axons, and wavy collagen fibres.

QUESTION 83

Which is the odd one out?

4 Vitiligo and poliosis

These occur in Vogt–Harada–Koyanagi syndrome; all other conditions may be found in sarcoidosis.

Lupus pernio is characterized by indurated, violaceous skin lesions on exposed parts of the body such as the cheeks (**1**), nose, fingers or ears. Bilateral **hilar adenopathy** (**2**) occurs in acute-onset sarcoid and may form part of Lofgren syndrome which also manifests erythema nodosum, often accompanied by fever and/or arthralgia. Cranial nerve palsy, often **facial** (**3**) is a feature of Heerfordt syndrome (uveoparotid fever) together with uveitis, parotid gland enlargement and fever. **Histology** in sarcoidosis shows non-caseating granulomatous inflammation (**5**). **Lacrimal gland** involvement (**6**) may result in keratoconjunctivitis sicca.

QUESTION 84

What are these juxtalimbal lesions?

1. Epithelial (racial) melanosis is characterized by flat, patchy, brownish pigmentation scattered throughout the conjunctiva but more intensely at the limbus.

2. Primary conjunctival melanoma appears as a black or grey nodule with dilated feeder vessels, most commonly located at the limbus but may arise anywhere in the conjunctiva. Conjunctival melanoma may also arise from primary acquired melanosis with atypia, and rarely from a pre-existing naevus.

3. Conjunctival papillomas, which may be multiple, are most frequent located in the juxtalimbal area, fornix or caruncle. Small lesions may not require treatment because they often resolve spontaneously. Large lesions are treated by excision or cryotherapy. Treatment options for recurrences include subconjunctival alpha-interferon, topical mitomycin C or oral cimetidine (Tagamet).

4. Ciliary body melanoma may extend through the emissary vessels and appear as a black epibulbar mass.

5. Nodular squamous cell carcinoma is a fleshy, pink papillomatous mass with feeder vessels often at the limbus but may be anywhere. Well-differentiated lesions grow slowly and may have a leukoplakia appearance. Metastasis can rarely occur to regional lymph nodes and systemically.

6. Dermoid is a smooth, soft, yellowish lesion, most frequently located at the infero-temporal limbus. Occasionally the lesions are very large and may virtually encircle the limbus (complex choristoma). Systemic associations include Goldenhar syndrome, and less commonly Treacher–Collins syndrome, and naevus sebaceus syndrome of Jadassohn.

QUESTION 85

What are these?

1. Cosmetic anterior chamber intraocular implant.

2. Corneal tattoo for cosmetic reasons.

3. Keratoprosthesis is an artificial corneal implant used in patients unsuitable for keratoplasty. The modern osteo-odonto-keratoprosthesis consists of the patient's own tooth root and alveolar bone which supports the central optical cylinder. This is usually covered with a buccal mucous membrane graft. Surgery is difficult and time consuming and is performed in two stages 2–4 months apart.

4. Ptosis props attached to spectacles.

5. Ptosis prop contact lens.

6. Artificial iris implant for aniridia.

QUESTION 86

Which of these require treatment?

1. Degenerative retinoschisis with breaks in the inner layer does not require treatment because the risk of retinal detachment is extremely low as there is no communication between the vitreous cavity and the subretinal space.

2. Pavingstone degeneration is characterized by discrete yellow-white patches of focal chorioretinal

atrophy. It is innocuous and is present to some extent in 25% of normal eyes.

3. Lattice degeneration is present in about 8% of the population. It is found more commonly in moderate myopes and is the most important degeneration directly related to retinal detachment. It is characterized by spindle-shaped areas of retinal thinning, most frequently located between the equator and the posterior border of the vitreous base. A characteristic feature is an arborizing network of white lines within the islands. Prophylactic treatment is usually reserved for fellow eyes of patients with retinal detachment.

4. Honeycomb (reticular) degeneration is an innocuous age-related change characterized by a fine network of perivascular pigmentation which may extend posterior to the equator.

5. Large superior U-tear with shallow surrounding subretinal fluid should be treated without delay to prevent extension of the detachment to involve the macula. Treatment involves local scleral buckling and cryotherapy.

6. White-with-pressure is frequently seen in normal eyes and does not require treatment.

QUESTION 87

What procedures were responsible for these complications?

1. Cataract surgery. Delayed-onset endophthalmitis occurs when an organism of low virulence becomes trapped within the capsular bag. It has an onset ranging from 4 weeks to years (mean of 9 months) post-operatively and typically follows uneventful surgery. An enlarging capsular plaque composed of organisms sequestrated in residual cortex within the peripheral capsular bag is characteristic.

2. Phacoemulsification which has damaged the inferior iris, probably when surgery was performed in the presence of a small pupil.

3. Steroid injection of periorbital capillary haemangioma. The injection was inadvertently intra-arterial and resulted in severe necrosis of the scalp and loss of the globe.

4. Cataract surgery. Dislocation of fragments of lens material into the vitreous cavity after zonular dehiscence or posterior capsule rupture is rare but potentially serious because it may result in glaucoma, chronic uveitis, retinal detachment, and chronic cystoid macular oedema. Initially uveitis or raised intraocular pressure must be treated. The patient should then be referred to a vitreoretinal surgeon for removal of nuclear fragments by pars plana vitrectomy.

5. Ganciclovir slow-release device (Vitrasert) is as effective as intravenous therapy in the treatment of cytomegalovirus retinitis. The duration of efficacy is 8 months, which is superior to intravenous therapy with either ganciclovir or foscarnet (average 60 days). However, it does not prevent involvement of the fellow eye. Complications include cataract (as in this case), vitreous haemorrhage, retinal detachment, and endophthalmitis.

6. Brachytherapy with radioactive plaques is frequently used to treat choroidal melanomas. Complications depend on the size of the tumour and its distance from optic nerve and fovea. Radiation retinopathy may develop 2–3 years after treatment. It is characterized by oedema, hard exudates, retinal capillary closure, telangiectasis, and neovascularization.

Match the angiogram (1–3) with the OCT (A–C)

I and B

Central serous retinopathy. FA shows upward flow of dye within the area of serous detachment (**1**). OCT shows separation of the sensory retina from the RPE (**B**).

2 and A

Detachment of the RPE. ICG shows a circular area of hyperfluorescence surrounded by a faint ring of hyperfluorescence (**2**). OCT shows separation of the RPE from Bruch membrane (**A**).

3 and C

Cystoid macular oedema. FA shows hyperfluorescence at the posterior pole that has a central 'flower-petal' appearance (**3**). OCT shows increased retinal thickness and intraretinal cystoid spaces (**C**).

What are the underlying causes of the cotton-wool spots?

1. Pre-proliferative diabetic retinopathy is caused by progressive retinal ischaemia. It is characterized by cotton-wool spots, intraretinal microvascular abnormalities (IRMA), which are arteriolar-venular shunts that run from retinal arterioles to venules, venous changes (dilatation, tortuosity, looping, and beading), arteriolar narrowing, and dark blot haemorrhages.

SECTION 2 ANSWERS

149

2. Papilloedema, when well developed, is characterized by swelling of the optic nerve head and peripapillary cotton-wool spots. Both eyes are invariably involved.

3. Retinal branch vein occlusion manifests dilatation and tortuosity of the venous segment distal to the site of occlusion and attenuation proximal to the occlusion, flame-shaped and dot-blot haemorrhages, retinal oedema, and sometimes cotton-wool spots in the sector of the retina drained by the obstructed vein.

4. Malignant hypertension is characterized by swelling of the optic nerve head, flame-shaped haemorrhages, a macular star, and scattered cotton-wool spots.

5. Purtscher retinopathy is caused by microvascular damage associated with severe trauma, especially to the head, and compressive chest injury. Other causes include embolism (fat, air or amniotic fluid) and a variety of systemic diseases. Cases not associated with trauma are sometimes referred to as 'Purtscher-like retinopathy'. The fundus shows multiple, unilateral or bilateral, superficial, white retinal patches resembling large cotton-wool spots, often associated with superficial peripapillary haemorrhages.

6. Leukaemic retinopathy is characterized by retinal haemorrhages, cotton-wool spots, which are probably caused by vascular occlusion by leukaemic cells, and retinal haemorrhages with white centres (Roth spots) composed either of leukaemic cells or platelet-fibrin emboli.

QUESTION 90

What are these complications of penetrating keratoplasty?

1. Infectious keratitis of the donor is uncommon. Risk factors include persistent epithelial defects, use of contact lenses, topical steroid therapy, loose or broken sutures, and keratoconjunctivitis sicca.

2. Acute bacterial endophthalmitis is less common than that following cataract surgery. Contaminated donor tissue or corneal storage media may be the source of the infection.

3. Rejection of the graft is frequently preceded by ciliary injection and anterior uveitis with keratic precipitates on the graft. Rejection may involve the epithelium, stroma or endothelium. The latter is the most severe because it can lead to endothelial cell loss and decompensation.

4. Epithelial ingrowth is a rare complication of anterior segment surgery in which conjunctival or corneal epithelial cells migrate through the wound and proliferate in the anterior segment, in a cystic or diffuse manner. The latter is characterized by the proliferation of sheets of epithelial cells over the posterior cornea, trabeculum, iris, and ciliary body, and is more commonly associated with secondary glaucoma than the cystic variety.

5. Persistent epithelial defects may lead to graft failure because re-epithelialization and maintenance of an intact epithelium is critical. Epithelial defects are most likely to occur in patients with pre-existing ocular surface disease such as alkali burns, neurotrophic keratopathy, and cicatrizing conjunctivitis.

6. Suture exposure may result in ocular irritation, corneal vascularization, and irritation of the superior tarsal conjunctiva, resulting in giant papillary conjunctivitis.

QUESTION 91

What are these ocular imaging techniques?

1. A-scan ultrasonography is performed with a single ultrasound source. It produces a one-dimensional time-amplitude evaluation in the form of vertical spikes along a baseline. The height of the spikes is proportional to the strength of the echo. The greater the distance to the right, the greater the distance between the source of the sound and the reflecting surface. The distance between individual spikes can be precisely measured. It is used mainly to measure anterior chamber depth, lens thickness, and axial length.

2. B-scan ultrasonography may be performed with a vector probe or a linear probe. The amount of reflected sound is portrayed as a dot of light. The more sound reflected, the brighter the dot. It provides topographic information concerning the size, shape, and quality of a lesion as well as its relationship to other structures. Moderate frequency (7–10 MHz) ultrasonography is used to examine the globe. The main indications are: evaluation of eyes with opaque media for retinal detachment, evaluation of posterior intraocular tumours, and detection of calcification as in retinoblastoma and optic disc drusen. Low frequency transducers (2–5 MHz) allow orbital examination.

3. High frequency ultrasonography utilizes 30–50 MHz that provides high-definition imaging of the anterior segment but only to a depth of 5 mm. It is of particular value in the evaluation of the anterior chamber in eyes with congenital corneal opacification.

4. Fluorescein angiography (FA) involves photographic surveillance of the passage of fluorescein through the retinal and choroidal circulations following intravenous injection. Fluorescence is the property of certain molecules to emit light of a longer wavelength when stimulated by light of a shorter wavelength. The excitation peak for fluorescein is about 490 nm (blue part of the spectrum) and represents the maximal absorption of light energy by fluorescein. Molecules stimulated by this wavelength will be excited to a higher energy level and will emit light of a longer wavelength at about 530 nm (green part of the spectrum). The angiogram consists of the following overlapping phases: choroidal (pre-arterial), arterial, arteriovenous (capillary), venous, and late (elimination). FA is used mainly to study the retinal circulation and the diagnosis of macular disease.

5. Optical coherence tomography (OCT) is a non-invasive, non-contact imaging system which provides high resolution cross-sectional images of the retina, vitreous, and optic nerve. OCT is analogous to B-scan ultrasonography but uses light instead of sound waves. Cross-sectional images are generated by scanning the optical beam in the transverse direction, thus yielding a two-dimensional data set that can be displayed as a false-colour or greyscale image. The main use of OCT is in the diagnosis or monitoring of macular pathology such as holes, cystoid oedema, epiretinal membranes, vitreomacular traction, and central serous retinopathy.

6. Indocyanine green (ICG) angiography is of particular value in studying the choroidal circulation and can be a useful adjunct to FA in the investigation of macular disease.

QUESTION 92

What has caused these inferior forniceal conditions?

1. Bacterial conjunctivitis is characterized by diffuse conjunctival injection most intense in the fornices and a papillary reaction over the tarsal conjunctiva. Initially the discharge is watery and then becomes mucopurulent.

2. Stevens–Johnson syndrome may cause conjunctival scarring and keratinization, and posterior lid margin disease with opening of meibomian gland orifices onto the eyelid surface.

3. Melanoma arising from primary acquired melanosis is characterized by irregular areas of flat, brown conjunctival pigmentation within which develop black areas of thickening and nodularity.

4. Chalazion granuloma is caused by rupture of the lesion through the tarsal conjunctiva.

5. Sporotrichosis is caused by the fungus *Sporothrix schenckii* that typically causes cutaneous infection. It can also cause a granulomatous conjunctivitis, as well as eyelid and orbital infection.

6. Conjunctival varices are uncommon and usually co-exist with orbital lesions. They characteristically increase in size with the Valsalva manoeuvre.

QUESTION 93

What are these multiple signs?

1. Central retinal vein occlusion and **branch arterial occlusion**.

2. Branch retinal artery occlusion and **choroidal naevus**.

3. Deep retinal haemorrhages and **angioid streaks.** Because an eye with angioid streaks is fragile, relatively mild ocular trauma may result in choroidal rupture and subretinal bleeding.

4. Toxoplasma retinitis and **branch retinal artery occlusion** by the primary focus is uncommon but devastating.

5. Central retinal vein occlusion and **frosted branch angiitis.** The latter is characterized by florid translucent retinal perivascular sheathing of both arterioles and venules. It is usually bilateral, and may represent a rare specific syndrome (primary form), or more frequently, a common immune pathway in response to multiple infective agents. Retinal vein occlusion may occur in severe cases.

6. Preretinal haemorrhage and **macular hole** caused by blunt trauma.

QUESTION 94

What are these tests?

1. Confrontation using a hat pin can be used to test the peripheral visual field and also to detect gross central defects. The pin is held behind the patient's head and then slowly brought forward in an arc until it is perceived. This is performed in the four quadrants.

2. Finger-counting is a quick test for the detection of hemianopia and quadrantanopia due to neurological disease. Initially the patient is asked to identify the number of fingers presented in each quadrant. If this is normal the simultaneous finger counting test is performed to detect the phenomenon of 'extinction' in which the defective hemifield appears intact when tested alone, but when tested with simultaneous stimuli a subtle defect may be uncovered. The test is performed by asking the patient to count the number of fingers presented simultaneously in the two hemifields.

3. Lacrimal probing and irrigation are performed with a gently curved, blunt tipped lacrimal cannula on a 2 ml saline-filled syringe which is inserted into the lower punctum and advanced a few mm following the contour of the canaliculus prior to irrigation. The cannula can come either to a hard stop or a soft stop. A hard stop occurs if the cannula enters the lacrimal sac. A soft stop is experienced if the cannula stops at or proximal to the junction of the common canaliculus and the lacrimal sac.

4. Exophthalmometry with a Hertel exophthalmometer is used to assess the severity of proptosis. The corneal apices are visualized in the mirrors and the degree of ocular protrusion is read off a scale. Readings greater than 20 mm are indicative of proptosis and a difference of 2 mm between the two eyes is suspicious regardless of the absolute value. Proptosis is graded as mild (21–23 mm), moderate (24–27 mm), and severe (28 mm or more).

5. The forced duction test is used to differentiate a restrictive from a neurological motility defect. After topical anaesthesia, the insertion of the muscle is grasped with forceps and the globe is rotated in the direction of limited mobility. Difficulty or inability to move the globe indicates a restrictive problem such as thyroid myopathy or muscle entrapment in an orbital floor fracture. Lack of resistance indicates a neurological paretic lesion.

6. Schirmer test is a useful assessment of aqueous tear production. The test involves measuring the amount of wetting of a special (no. 41 Whatman) filter paper. After 5 minutes the filter paper is removed and the amount of wetting from the fold measured. Less than 10 mm of wetting after 5 minutes without anaesthesia and less than 6 mm with anaesthesia is considered abnormal.

QUESTION 95

What are these subtle conditions?

1. Orbital varices causing a deep left superior sulcus due to fat atrophy. Orbital varices cause intermittent proptosis which is non-pulsatile and is not associated with a bruit. The proptosis may be precipitated or accentuated by increasing venous pressure through coughing, straining, Valsalva manoeuvre, assuming the dependent position or external compression of the jugular veins. Patients with long-standing lesions may develop atrophy of surrounding fat and enophthalmos associated with a deepened superior sulcus in the resting position, reversible with increase in venous pressure.

2. Superficial dermoid cyst in the supero-nasal part of the orbit. A dermoid cyst is a choristoma derived from displacement of ectoderm to a subcutaneous location along embryonic lines of closure. Dermoids may be superficial or deep to the orbital septum. Superficial dermoids are more commonly located supero-temporally than supero-nasally.

3. Benign mixed-cell tumour causing fullness in right supero-lateral region and mild mechanical ptosis. Pleomorphic adenoma (benign mixed-cell tumour) is the most common epithelial tumour of the lacrimal gland and is derived from the ducts and secretory elements including myoepithelial cells. Presentation is in the second to fifth decade with a painless, slowly progressive proptosis or swelling in the supero-lateral part of the orbit, usually of more than a year's duration.

4. Frontal mucocele causing slight left proptosis and downward displacement of the globe. A mucocele develops when the drainage of normal paranasal sinus secretions is obstructed due to infection, allergy, trauma, tumour or congenital narrowing. A slowly expanding cystic accumulation of mucoid secretions and epithelial debris develops and gradually erodes the bony walls of the sinuses, causing symptoms by encroaching upon surrounding tissues.

5. Chronic dacryocystitis causing a painless swelling in the inner canthus due to a mucocele. Obvious swelling may be absent, although pressure over the sac commonly results in reflux of mucopurulent material through the canaliculi.

6. Left facial palsy and **lateral tarsorrhaphy**, which has been performed to protect the cornea because of poor eyelid closure.

QUESTION 96

What are these ocular motility defects?

1. Duane retraction syndrome type 1. Eyes are straight in the primary position (**A**). Attempted left gaze shows gross limitation of left abduction with slight widening of the left palpebral fissure (**B**). Right gaze shows slight limitation of left adduction and return of left palpebral fissure to its normal position (**C**). In Duane retraction syndrome there is failure of innervation of the lateral rectus by the sixth nerve, with anomalous innervation by fibres from the third nerve. The condition is often bilateral, although fre-

quently involvement of the other eye may be very subtle. Some children have associated congenital defects such as perceptive deafness and speech disorder.

2. Convergence excess esotropia. Eyes are straight in the primary position (**A**); gross right esotropia for near (**B**); straight eyes when looking through reading segment of bifocals (**C**). Non-refractive accommodative esotropia is associated with a high AC/A ratio in which a unit increase of accommodation is accompanied by a disproportionately large increase of convergence. This occurs independently of refractive error, although hypermetropia frequently co-exists. In convergence excess the high AC/A ratio is due to increased accommodative convergence (accommodation is normal, convergence is increased).

QUESTION 97

Match the fundus (1–3) with the scan (A–C)

1 and C

Raised intracranial pressure is characterized by papilloedema (**1**) and dilated ventricles (hydrocephalus – **C**). Papilloedema is invariably bilateral although it may be asymmetrical in severity. In communicating hydrocephalus the CSF flows from the ventricular system to the subarachnoid space without impediment. The obstruction to flow lies in the basilar cisterns or in the subarachnoid space, where there is failure of absorption by the arachnoid villi. Non-communicating hydrocephalus is caused by obstruction to CSF flow in the ventricular system or at the exit foramina of the fourth ventricle. The CSF therefore does not have access to the subarachnoid space.

2 and B

Multiple sclerosis may cause retrobulbar neuritis which is characterized by visual loss in the presence of a normal optic nerve head (**2**). At the first episode of retrobulbar neuritis patients who also show T2-weighted periventricular lesions on MR (**B**) but no clinical evidence of demyelination, have a 56% risk of developing multiple sclerosis within 10 years.

3 and A

Von Hippel–Lindau syndrome is an AD phacomatosis characterized by retinal haemangioblastomas (**3**), and a variety of systemic tumours and cystic lesions. CNS haemangioblastoma involving the cerebellum (**A**), spinal cord, medulla or pons affects about 25% of patients with retinal tumours. Conversely about 50% of patients with solitary retinal lesions and virtually all patients with multiple lesions have von Hippel–Lindau syndrome.

3. Lepromatous iritis may result in iris atrophy and miosis as a result of damage to the sympathetic innervation to the dilator pupillae.

4. Fuchs uveitis syndrome results in stromal iris atrophy that renders the sphincter pupillae more prominent.

5. Rieger anomaly is a bilateral congenital condition characterized by variable stromal hypoplasia, which may be associated with ectropion uveae, corectopia, and pseudopolycoria. Glaucoma develops during early childhood in 50% of cases.

6. Severe blunt trauma may result in extensive disintegration of part of the iris and atrophy of the remainder.

QUESTION 98

What has caused these atrophic iris lesions?

1. Iridoschisis is a rare condition which typically affects the elderly and is often bilateral. It is associated with underlying angle-closure glaucoma in 90% of cases. It is thought that acute or intermittent angle closure results in iris atrophy because of high IOP. The iridoschisis usually involves the inferior iris and may range in severity from intrastromal atrophy to extensive splitting of the anterior leaf (**1**) with disintegrated iris fibrils.

2. Post-congestive angle closure is characterized by spiral-shaped iris atrophy and a fixed dilated pupil.

QUESTION 99

What systemic disease has caused these problems?

Diabetes mellitus

Monilial infection (**1**) is a common recurring problem. **Ocular motor nerve palsies**, particularly sixth (**2**) or a pupil sparing third may occur as a result of small vessel disease. **Degenerative arthropathy** (Charcot joints) as a result of sensory polyneuropathy (**3**). **Lipodystrophy** at sites of insulin injection (**4**). **Neuropathic ulceration** leading to painless perforating ulceration at pressure points on the soles (**5**). Diabetic mothers tend to give birth to **large babies** (**6**).

QUESTION 100

What do these angiograms show?

1. Old retinal branch vein occlusion. FA arterial phase shows mild hypofluorescence corresponding to the area drained by the vein as well as mild patchy hypofluorescence due to blockage by hard exudates and flame-shaped haemorrhages. Venous phase shows delayed venous filling, extensive hypofluorescence due to capillary dropout which also involves the foveal avascular zone, and 'pruning' of vessels. Late phase shows persistent hypofluorescence of the ischaemic area, and perivascular hyperfluorescence due to staining.

2. Proliferative diabetic retinopathy. FA arterial phase shows mild spotty hyperfluorescence temporal to the disc from microaneurysms, and two areas of hypofluorescence above due to blockage by flame-shaped haemorrhages. The venous phase highlights venous dilatation and beading and also shows extensive spotty hyperfluorescence at the posterior pole from microaneurysms and capillary abnormalities. There are also extensive areas of hypofluorescence due to capillary drop-out and a patch of hyperfluorescence at the disc indicative of early new vessel formation. Later phase shows extensive diffuse hyperfluorescence at the posterior pole due to leakage.

3. Disciform scarring and haemorrhage in myopia due to choroidal neovascularization resulting from either lacquer cracks or areas of patchy atrophy. FA shows extensive hypofluorescence due to blockage by blood, with a central area of increasing hyperfluorescence due to staining of the disciform scar.

4. Polypoidal choroidal vasculopathy (PCV) is a relatively uncommon, idiopathic choroidal vascular disease in which the inner choroidal vessels develop multiple terminal aneurysmal protuberances with a polypoidal configuration. The two main types are exudative and haemorrhagic. ICG is required to make a definitive diagnosis of PCV. This shows a branching vascular network from the choroidal circulation and polypoidal and aneurysmal dilatations at the terminals of the branching vessels that fill slowly and then leak intensely.

Section 3

Questions 101 to 150. Answers start on page 208.

Q 101 What have these conditions in common?

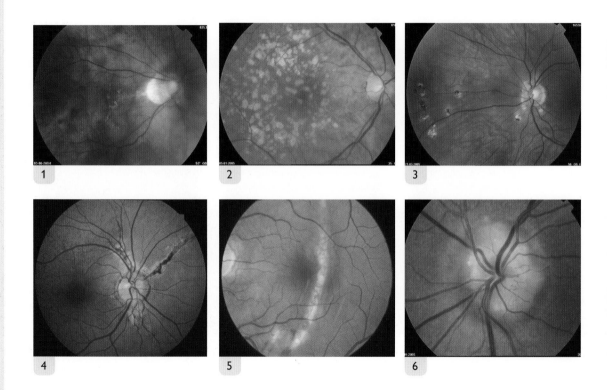

1

2

3

4

5

6

Answer on pages 208–209

Q **102** Benign or malignant?

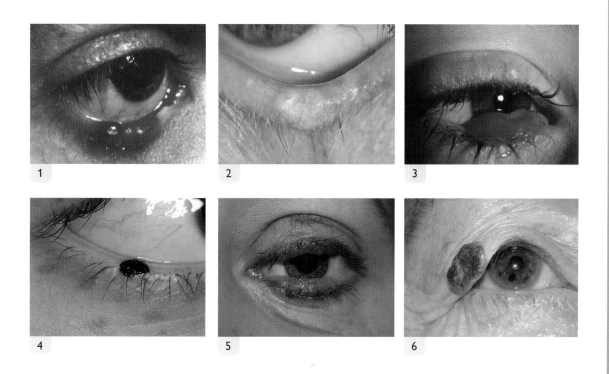

1

2

3

4

5

6

Answer on page 209

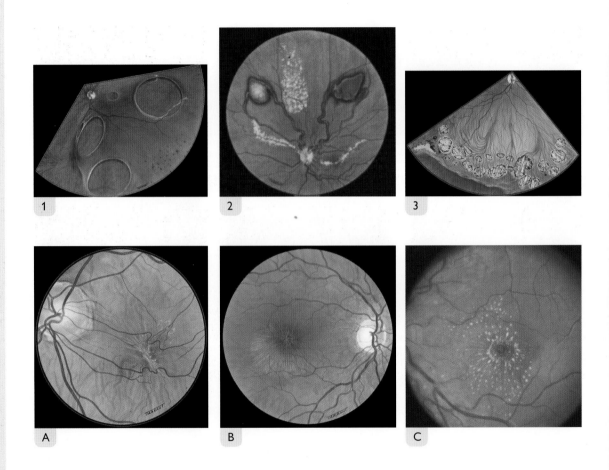

Q **103** Match the peripheral lesion (1–3) with the maculopathy (A–C)

Answer on pages 209–210

Q 104 What are these canthal lesions?

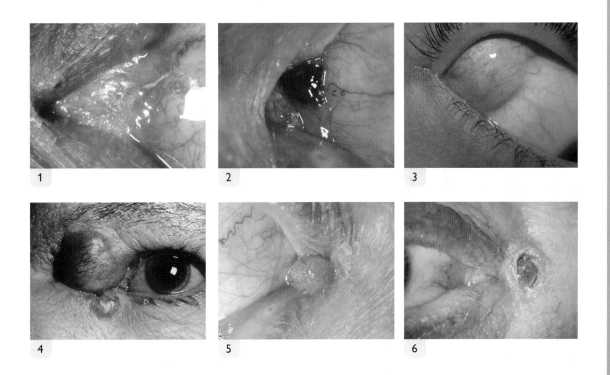

1

2

3

4

5

6

Answer on page 210

Q **105** What are the possible underlying causes?

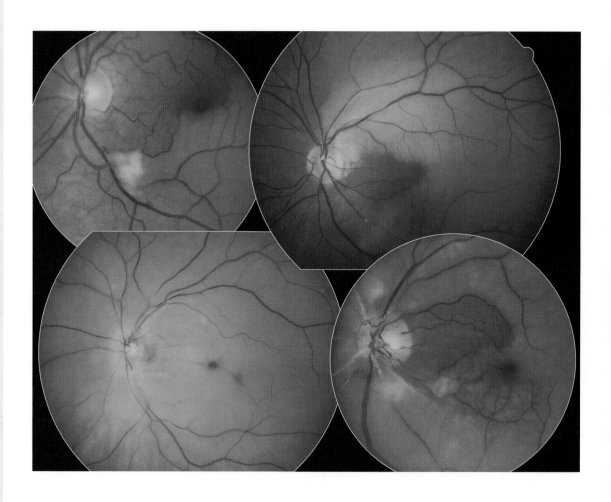

Answer on page 210

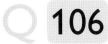
Q **106** What are the underlying metabolic disorders?

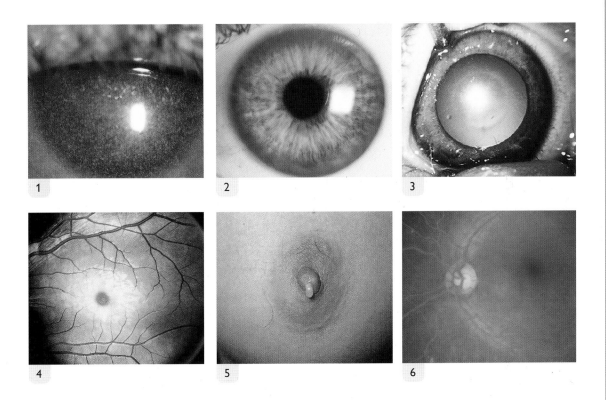

1

2

3

4

5

6

Answer on pages 210–211

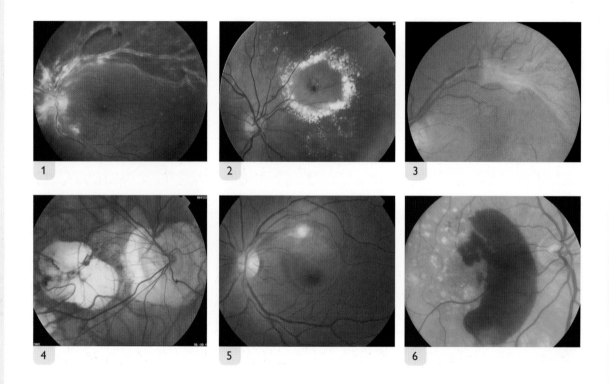

Answer on pages 211–212

Q 108   What pathogens are involved?

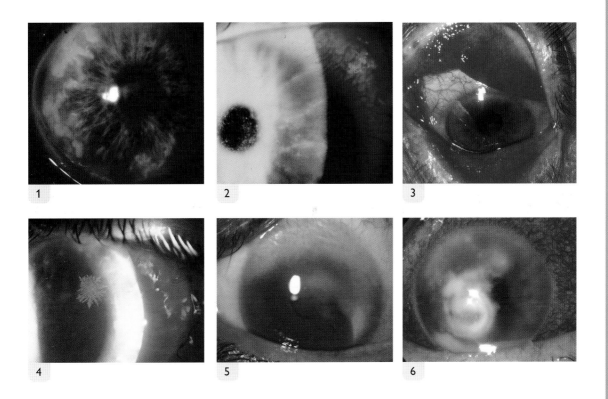

Answer on page 212

109 What treatment has been performed and for what reason?

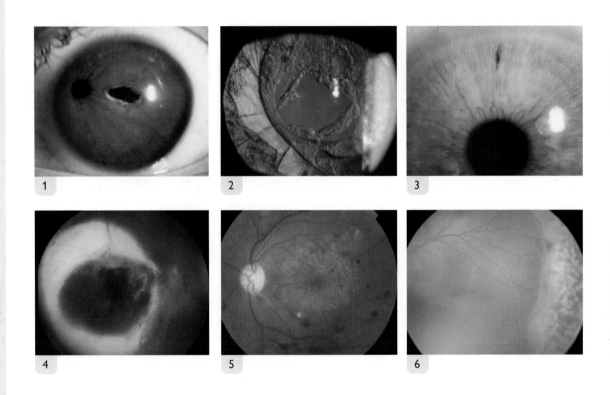

1

2

3

4

5

6

Answer on pages 212–213

Q 110 What are these complications of trabeculectomy?

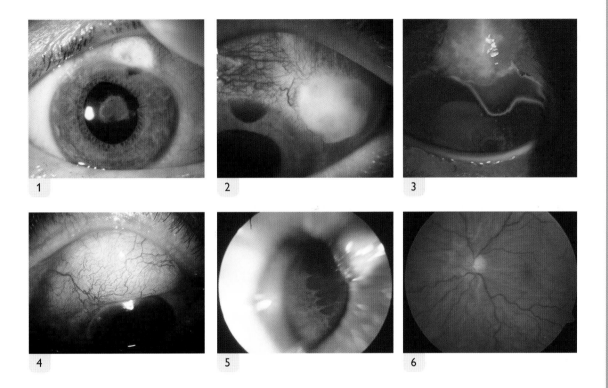

1

2

3

4

5

6

Answer on pages 213–214

Q 111 Match the skin (1–3) with the eye (A–C)

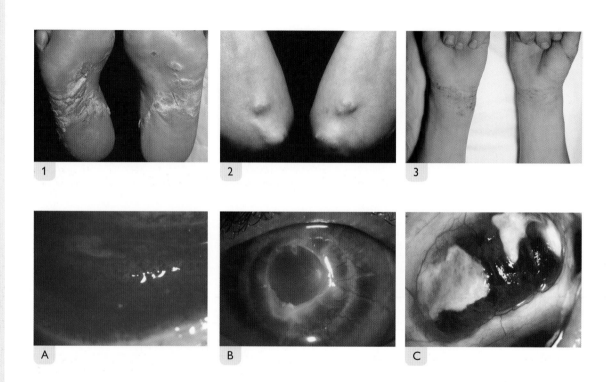

Answer on page 214

Q 112 Diabetic retinopathy – is treatment required?

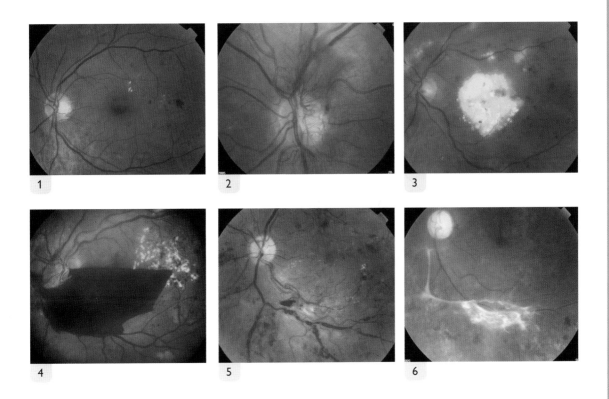

Answer on pages 214–215

Q **113** Match the orbital lesion (1–3) with the CT (A–C)

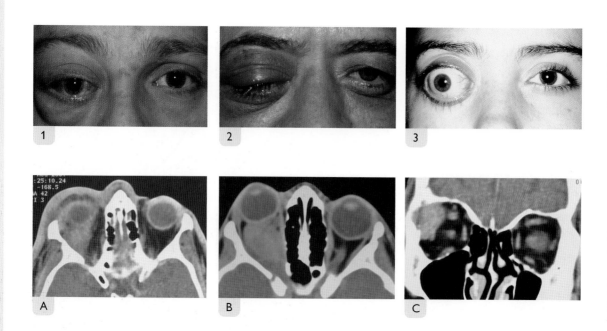

Answer on page 215

Q **114** What are these uncommon fundus conditions?

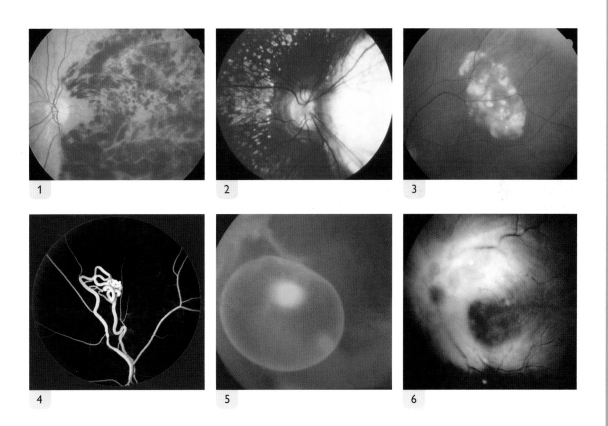

Answer on pages 215–216

171

Q 115 What are these ocular motility defects?

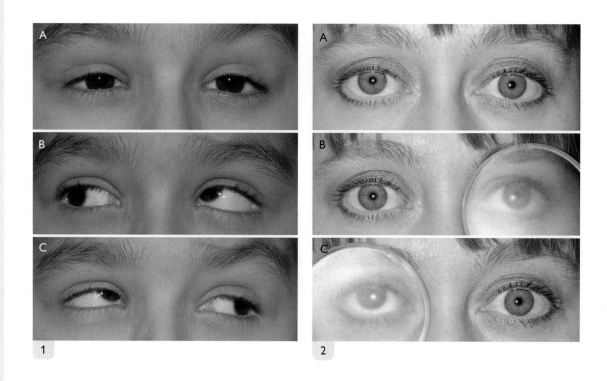

Answer on page 216

Q 116 What are these subtle signs?

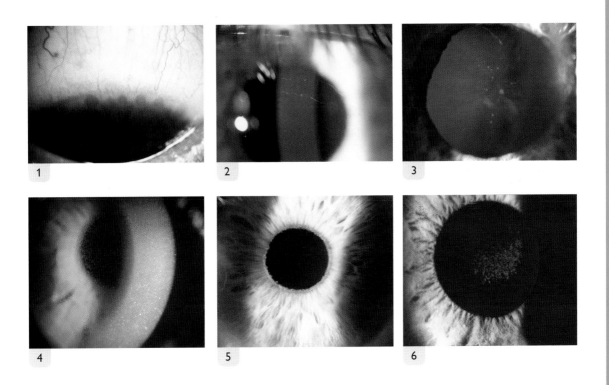

Answer on page 216

Q **117** What treatment is being performed?

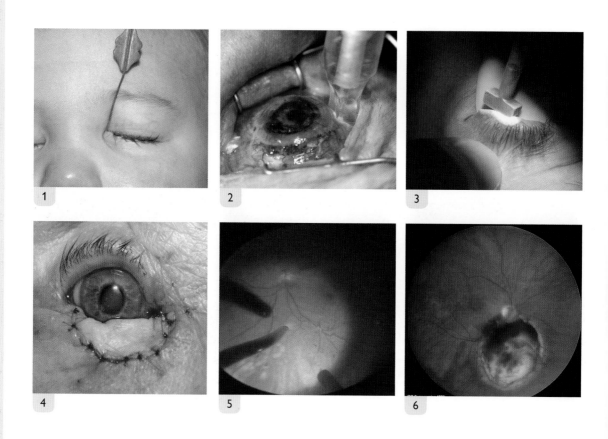

Answer on pages 216–217

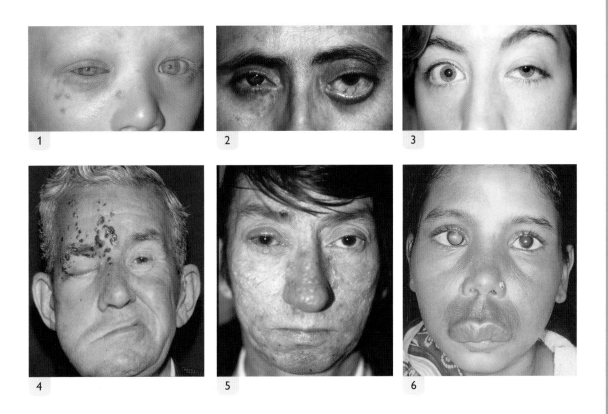

Q 118 What multiple signs do these patients show?

Answer on page 217

Q 119 Match the corneal dystrophy (1–3) with the stain (A–C)

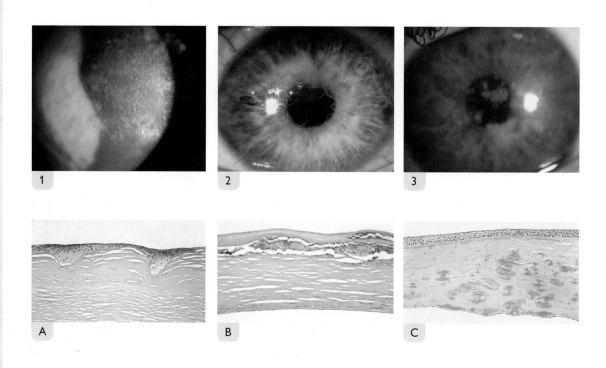

Answer on pages 217–218

Q 120 Which is the odd one out?

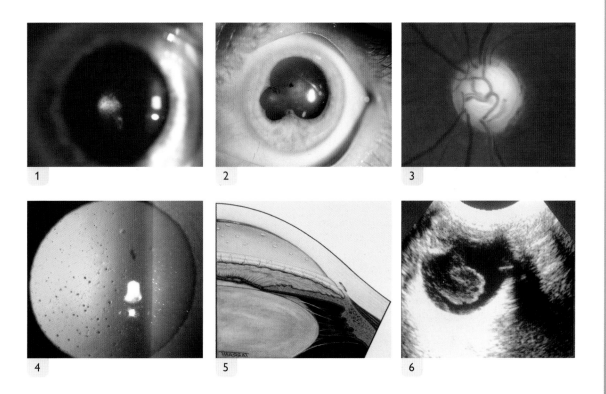

1

2

3

4

5

6

Answer on page 218

Q 121 What urinary abnormalities may be present?

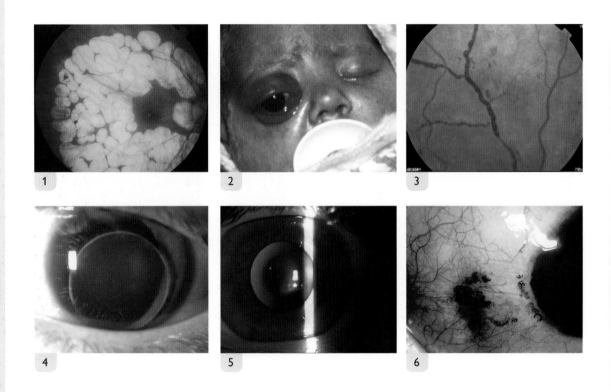

Answer on pages 218–219

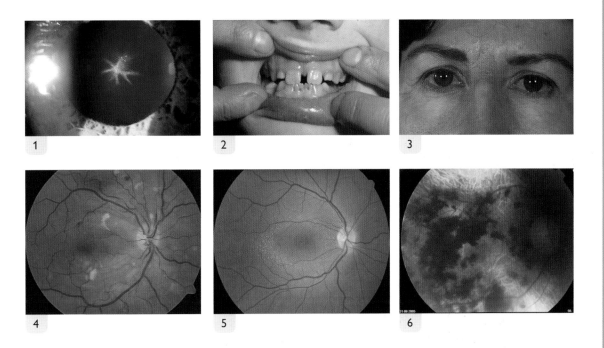

Answer on page 219

Q 123 Match (1) with one of (A–D)

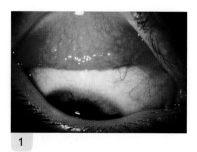

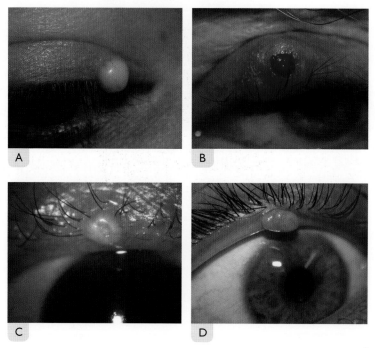

Answer on page 219

Q 124 Match the blood film (1–3) with the eye (A–C)

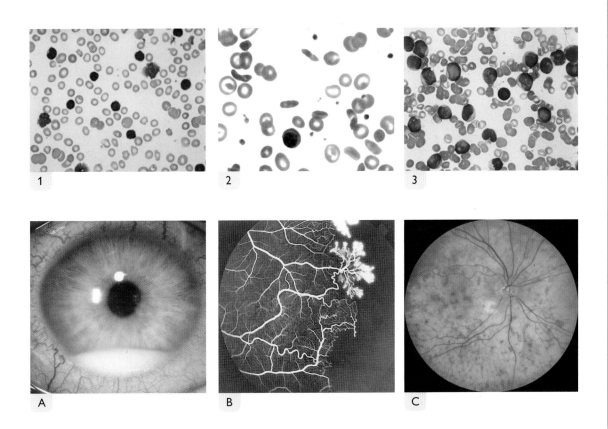

Answer on pages 219–220

Q 125 What do these fluorescein angiograms show?

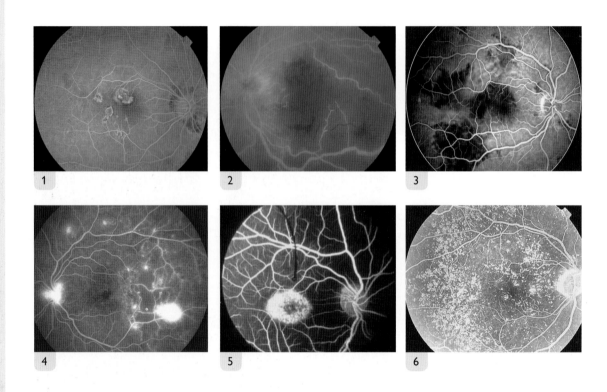

Answer on page 220

126 Hamartoma or choristoma?

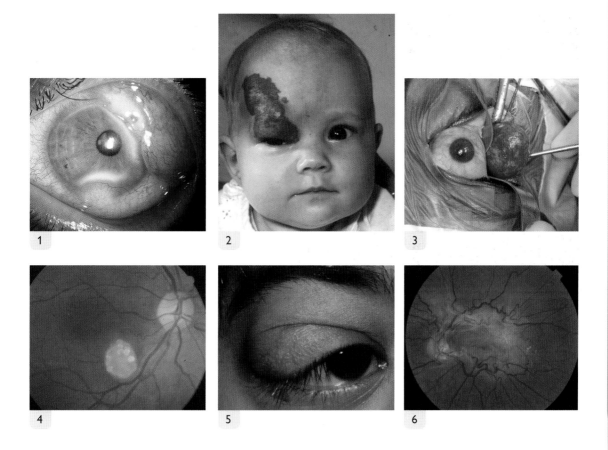

Answer on pages 220–221

Q 127 What do these charts show?

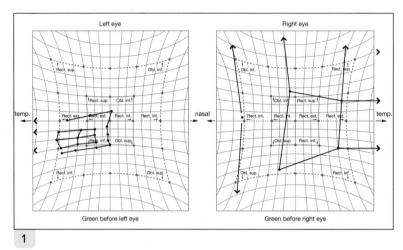

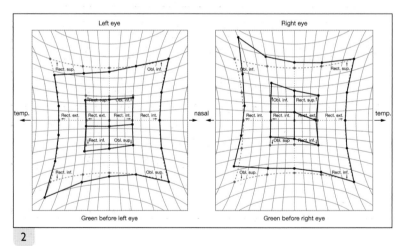

Answer on page 221

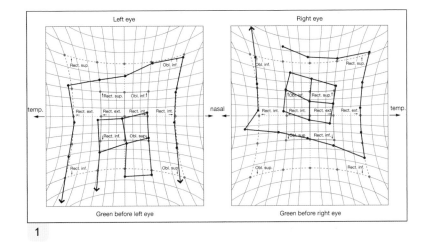

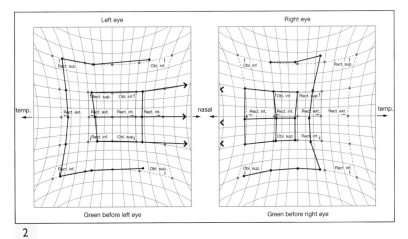

Q **128** What do these charts show?

1

2

Answer on pages 221–222

Q 129 What have these conditions in common?

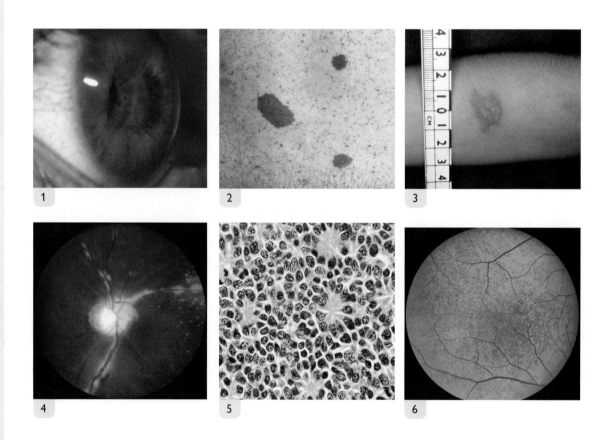

1

2

3

4

5

6

Answer on page 222

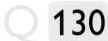
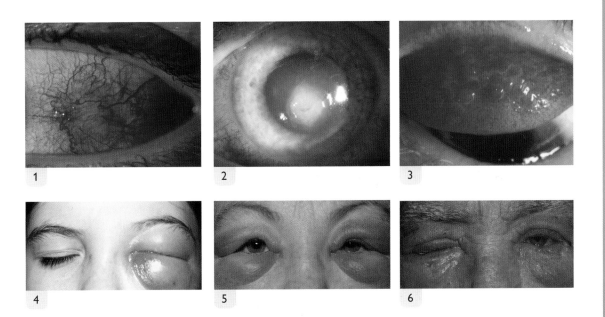

1

2

3

4

5

6

Answer on pages 222–223

Q 131 What are the HLA associations of these inflammatory conditions?

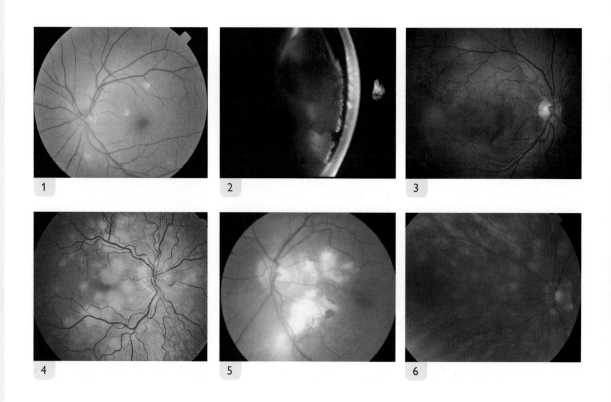

Answer on pages 223–224

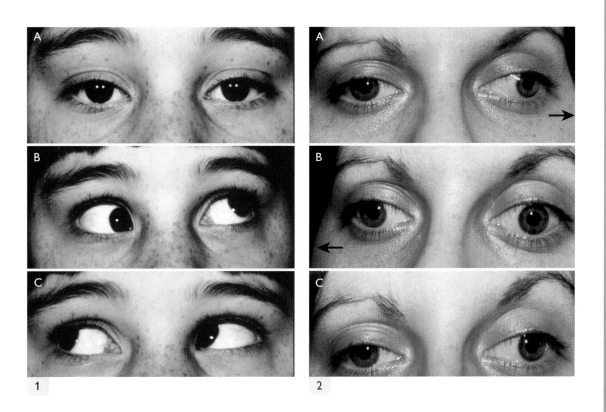

Q 132 What are these ocular motility defects?

Answer on page 224

189

Q 133 What are these subtle fundus lesions?

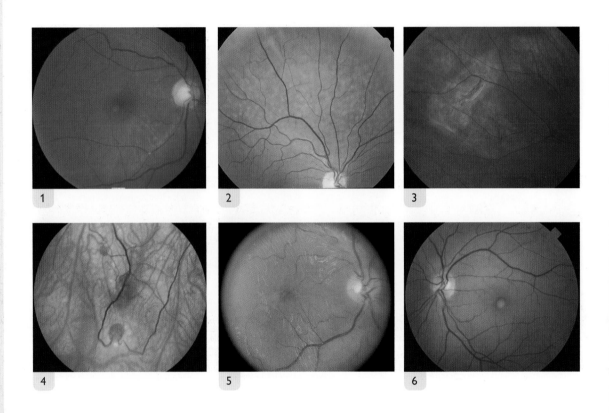

Answer on pages 224–225

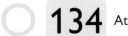

Q **134** At what age do these conditions present?

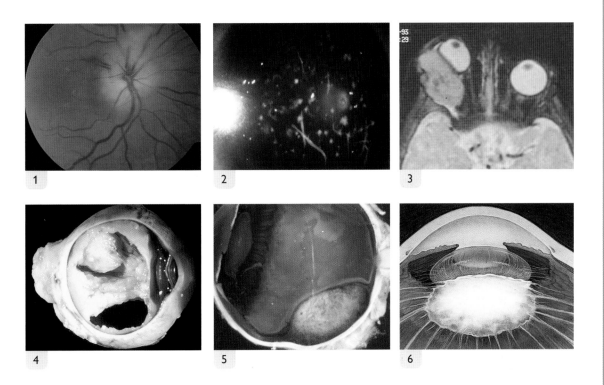

Answer on page 225

Q **135** What treatment has been performed?

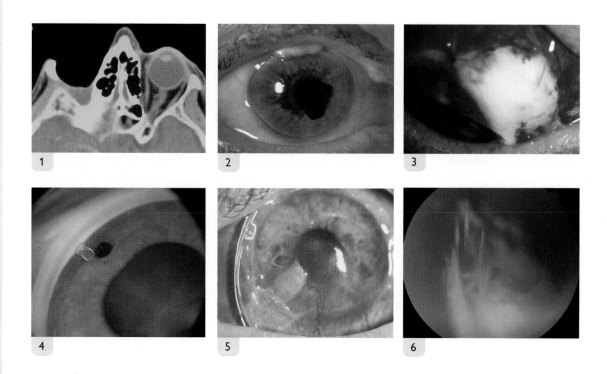

1

2

3

4

5

6

Answer on pages 225–226

Q 136 What have these conditions in common?

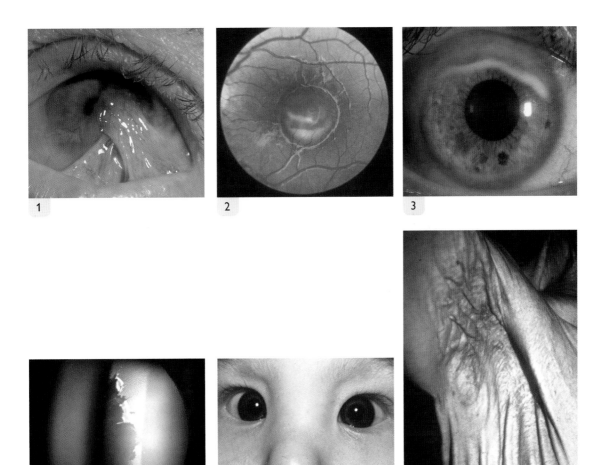

1

2

3

4

5

6

Answer on page 226

Q **137** What are the systemic associations of these conditions?

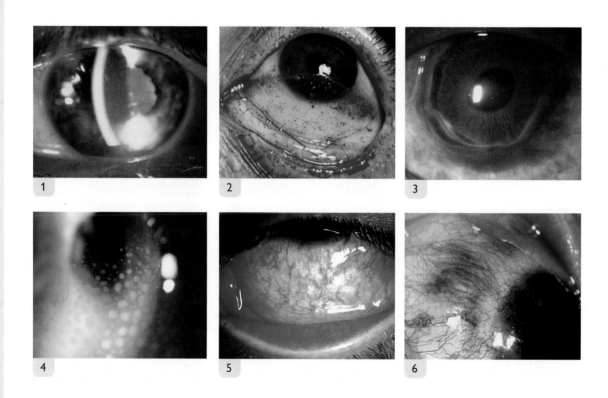

Answer on pages 226–227

138 Match the eye (1–3) with the histology (A–C)

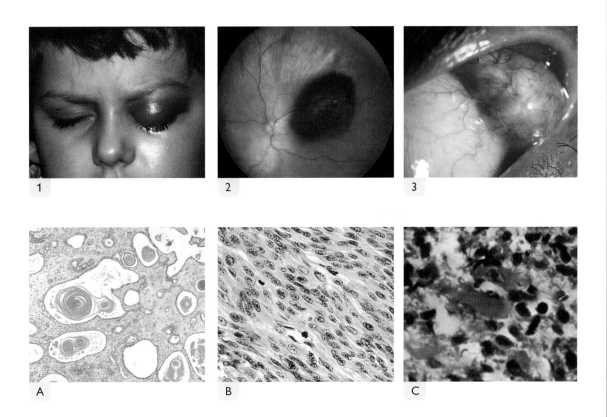

1

2

3

A

B

C

Answer on page 227

Match the fundus (1–3) with the gonioscopy (A–C)

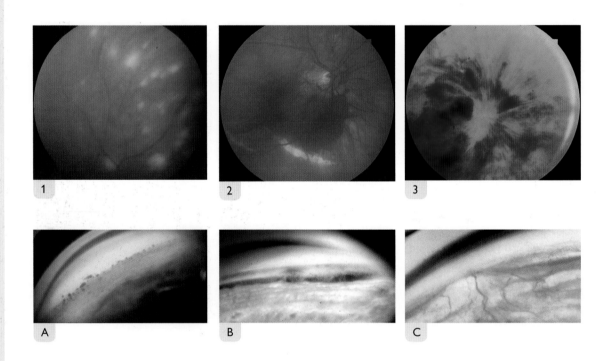

Answer on page 228

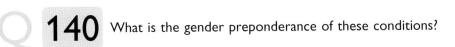

Q 140 What is the gender preponderance of these conditions?

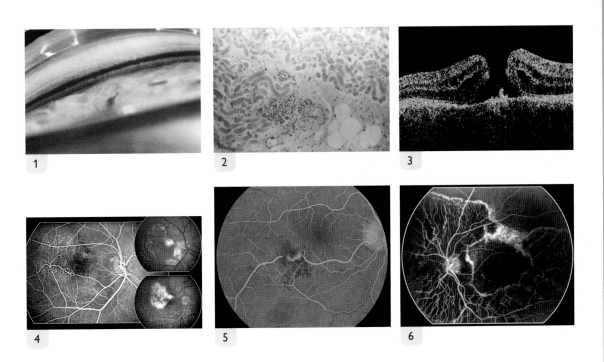

1

2

3

4

5

6

Answer on pages 228–229

Q 141 What is this disease?

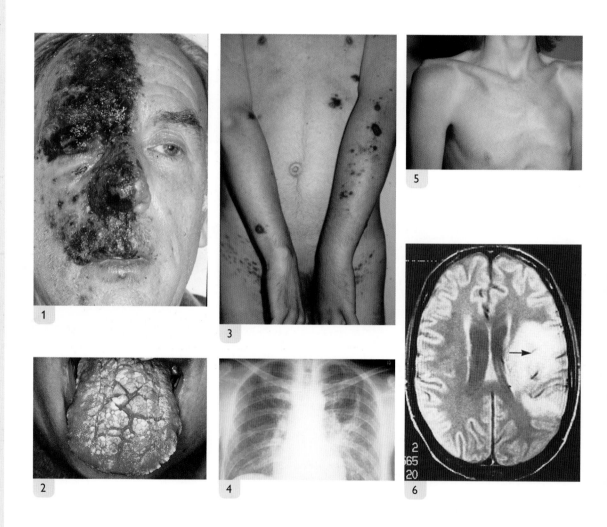

Answer on page 229

Q 142 At what level is the haemorrhage?

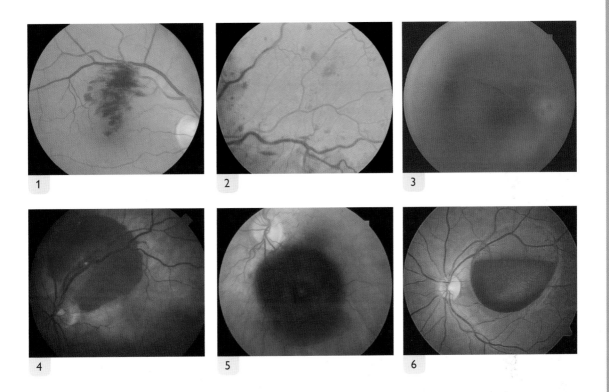

1

2

3

4

5

6

Answer on page 229

143 What multiple signs are present?

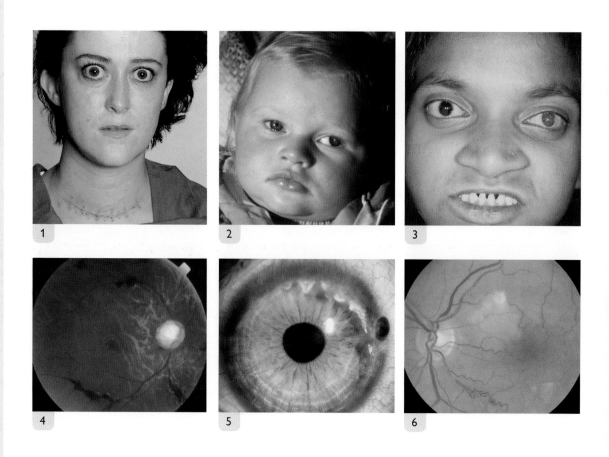

Answer on pages 229–230

Q **144** What have these conditions in common?

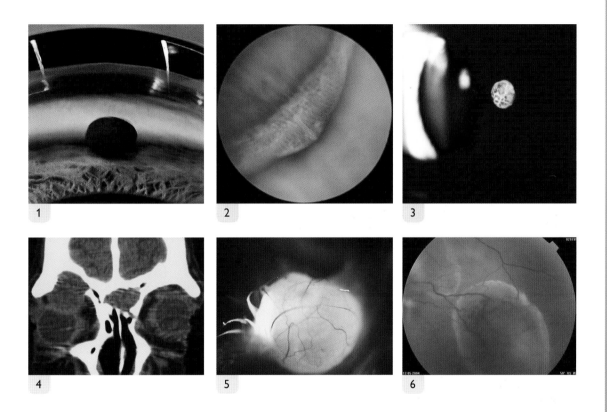

1

2

3

4

5

6

Answer on pages 230–231

Q **145** Which is the odd one out?

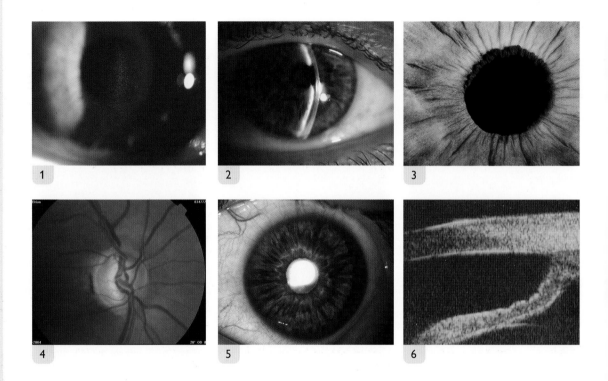

1

2

3

4

5

6

Answer on page 231

Q 146 Plant, fruit or mineral?

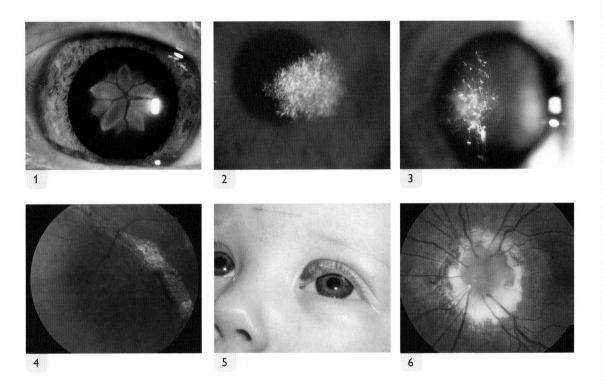

Answer on page 231

Q 147 What are these rare conditions?

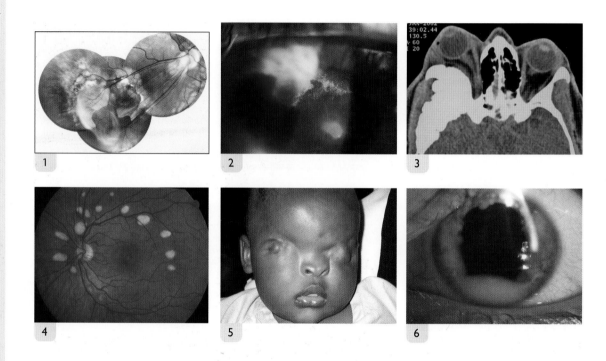

Answer on pages 231–232

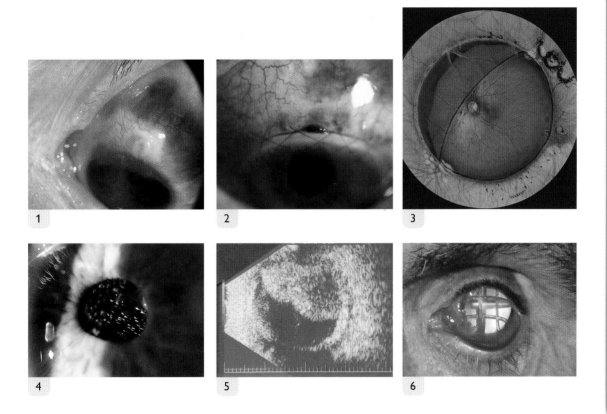

1 2 3

4 5 6

Answer on page 232

Q 149 What have these conditions in common?

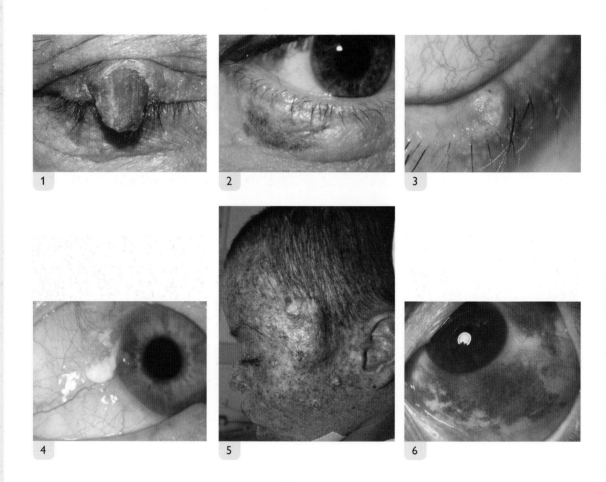

Answer on page 233

Q 150 Match the clinical sign (1–3) with the angiogram (A–C)

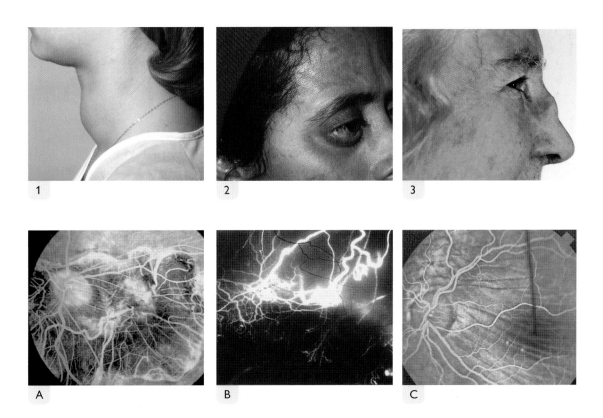

Answer on pages 233–234

QUESTION 101

What have these conditions in common?

They are all associated with choroidal neovascularization

1. Lacquer cracks in high myopia consist of ruptures in the RPE–Bruch membrane–choriocapillaris complex characterized clinically by fine, irregular, yellow lines, often branching and criss-crossing at the posterior pole. They are potentially sight-threatening as they may precede the development of choroidal neovascularization (CNV).

2. Drusen are yellow excrescences beneath the RPE, distributed symmetrically at both posterior poles. They may vary in number, size, shape, degree of elevation, and extent of associated RPE changes. Although many patients with drusen maintain normal vision throughout life, a significant number of elderly patients develop AMD which may be dry or wet. Features associated with an increased risk of subsequent visual loss include large soft and/or confluent drusen, and focal hyperpigmentation of the RPE, particularly if the other eye has already developed AMD.

3. Presumed ocular histoplasmosis (POHS) is thought to represent an immunologic mediated response in individuals previously exposed to the fungus *Histoplasma capsulatum*. Patients with POHS show an increased prevalence of HLA-B7 and HLA-DR2. The fundus shows peripapillary atrophy as well as atrophic 'histo' spots consisting of roundish, slightly irregular, yellowish-white lesions often associated with pigment clumps scattered in the mid-retinal periphery and posterior fundus. CNV develops in about 5% of eyes most frequently in association with an old macular 'histo spot'.

4. Angioid streaks are the result of crack-like dehiscences in thickened, calcified, and abnormally brittle collagenous and elastic portions of Bruch membrane. Fundoscopy shows linear, grey or dark-red linear lesions with irregular serrated edges that lie beneath the normal retinal blood vessels. They intercommunicate in a ring-like fashion around the optic disc and then radiate outwards from the peripapillary area. Visual loss occurs in about 70% of cases, most frequently as a result of CNV.

5. Choroidal rupture is caused by severe blunt trauma and involves the choroid, Bruch membrane, and RPE. An old rupture appears as a white crescent-shaped, vertical streak of exposed underlying sclera concentric with the optic disc. An uncommon late complication is CNV which may result in haemorrhage, scarring, and visual impairment.

6. Optic disc drusen (hyaline bodies) are composed of hyaline-like calcific material within the substance of the optic nerve head. They are present in about 0.3% of the population and are often bilateral. During the early teens drusen usually emerge at the surface of the disc as waxy pearl-like irregularities associated with anomalous disc vasculature. Juxtapapillary CNV is an uncommon complication.

QUESTION 102

Benign or malignant?

1. Malignant – Kaposi sarcoma is a vascular tumour which typically affects patients with the acquired immune deficiency syndrome (AIDS). Many patients have advanced systemic disease although in some instances the tumour may be the sole manifestation. It is characterized by a pink, red-violet to brown lesion, which may be mistaken for a haematoma or a naevus.

2. Malignant – basal cell carcinoma (BCC) is the most common human malignancy; 90% of cases occur in the head and neck and about 10% of these involve the eyelid. BCC is by far the most common malignant eyelid tumour accounting for 90% of all cases. Nodular BCC is a shiny, firm, pearly nodule with small dilated blood vessels on its surface.

3. Benign – pyogenic granuloma is a fast-growing proliferation of granulation tissue which is usually antedated by surgery, trauma or infection although some cases are idiopathic. It is characterized by a painful, rapidly growing, vascular polypoidal lesion that may bleed following relatively trivial trauma.

4. Malignant – melanoma rarely develops on the eyelids but is potentially lethal. Superficial spreading melanoma is characterized by a plaque with an irregular outline and variable pigmentation. Nodular melanoma is characterized by a blue-black nodule surrounded by normal skin.

5. Benign – a kissing (split) congenital melanocytic naevus is a rare condition that equally involves the upper and lower eyelids.

6. Benign – seborrhoeic keratosis (basal cell papilloma, senile verruca) is a common, slow-growing condition found on the face, trunk, and extremities of elderly individuals. It is characterized by a discrete, greasy, brown plaque with a friable verrucous surface and a 'stuck-on' appearance.

QUESTION 103

Match the peripheral lesion (1–3) with the maculopathy (A–C)

1 and B

Congenital retinoschisis is an XL condition caused by a defect in Muller cells resulting in splitting of the retinal nerve fibre layer from the rest of the sensory retina. **Peripheral schisis** affects 50% of patients and is characterized by oval defects predominantly in the inferotemporal quadrant (**1**). All patients also manifest **foveal schisis** which is characterized by tiny cystoid spaces with a 'bicycle-wheel' pattern of radial striae (**B**).

2 and C

Retinal haemangioblastoma is a rare sight-threatening tumour that may occasionally occur in isolation although about 50% of patients with solitary lesions and virtually all patients with multiple lesions have von Hippel–Lindau disease. It is characterized by a round orange-red mass with dilatation and tortuosity of the supplying artery and draining vein (**2**). Hard exudates may form around the tumour as well as at the **macula** (**C**).

3 and A

Peripheral retinal cryotherapy is performed as a prophylactic measure in eyes at risk from rhegmatogenous retinal detachment (**3**). A very rare complication is the development of **macular pucker** (**A**).

QUESTION 104

What are these canthal lesions?

1. Flattening of the plica and **keratinization of the caruncle** occur in ocular cicatricial pemphigoid which is a rare autoimmune mucocutaneous blistering disease that typically affects elderly individuals.

2. Naevus at the caruncle and **plica.** A conjunctival naevus is a solitary, sharply demarcated, flat or slightly elevated, pigmented lesion most frequently found in the juxtalimbal area. The second most common location is the plica and caruncle. Around puberty the naevus may enlarge and become more pigmented.

3. Lipodermoid is a soft, movable, subconjunctival mass most commonly located at the outer canthus. Excision should be avoided because it may be complicated by scarring, ptosis, dry eye, and ocular motility problems.

4. Carcinoma of lacrimal sac, although extremely rare, should be considered in the differential diagnosis of epiphora associated with a mass in the medial canthus.

5. Papilloma of the conjunctiva may be pedunculated or sessile. The most frequent locations are juxtalimbal, caruncular, and forniceal.

6. Basal cell carcinoma most frequently arises from the lower eyelid, followed in order of frequency by the medial canthus, upper eyelid, and lateral canthus.

QUESTION 105

What are the possible underlying causes?

Atherosclerosis-related thrombosis at the level of the lamina cribrosa is by far the most common underlying cause of central retinal artery occlusion, accounting for about 80% of cases. Another important cause is calcific embolism from an atheromatous plaque at the carotid bifurcation and less commonly from the aortic arch. Emboli composed of cholesterol (Hollenhorst plaques) are usually asymptomatic and those composed of fibrin-platelet may cause transient visual loss (amaurosis fugax) but rarely permanent occlusion. Rare causes of retinal artery occlusion include giant cell arteritis, cardiac embolism, periarteritis, thrombophilic disorders, and sickling haemoglobinopathies.

QUESTION 106

What are the underlying metabolic disorders?

1. Cystinosis is a rare, AR, metabolic disorder characterized by widespread tissue deposition of cystine crystals as a result of a defect in lysosomal transport. Keratopathy is present by 1 year of age and is characterized by progressive deposition of crystals in the conjunctiva and cornea which cause intense photophobia, blepharospasm, epithelial erosions, and visual disability.

2. Wilson disease (hepatolenticular degeneration) is caused by deficiency of caeruloplasmin resulting in widespread tissue deposition of copper. Keratopathy is present in nearly all patients and is very useful in diagnosis. It is characterized by a zone of copper granules in the peripheral part of Descemet membrane (Kayser–Fleischer ring) which change colour under different types of illumination. The deposits are preferentially distributed in the vertical meridian and may disappear with penicillamine therapy.

3. Galactosaemia involves severe impairment of galactose utilization caused by absence of the enzyme galactose-1-phosphate uridyl transferase (GPUT). Inheritance is AR. A central 'oil droplet' lens opacity develops within a few days or weeks of life in a large percentage of patients. The exclusion of galactose (in milk products) from the diet prevents the progression of cataract and may reverse early lens changes.

4. Sphingolipidoses are characterized by the progressive intracellular accretion of excessive quantities of certain glycolipids and phospholipids in various tissues of the body, including the retina. The lipids accumulate in the ganglion cell layer giving the retina a white appearance. Because ganglion cells are absent at the foveola, this area retains relative transparency and contrasts with the surrounding opaque retina giving rise to a 'cherry-red' spot.

5. Excessive prolactin secretion by a chromophobe adenoma (prolactinoma) may cause the infertility-amenorrhoea-galactorrhoea syndrome in women. In men it may result in hypogonadism, impotence, sterility, and occasionally gynaecomastia.

6. Hypertriglyceridaemia, if severe, may rarely give rise to lipaemia retinalis characterized by creamy white coloured retinal blood vessels. The visualization of high levels of chylomicrons in blood vessels accounts for the fundus appearance. Visual acuity is usually normal but ERG amplitude may be decreased.

QUESTION 107

What has caused these complications?

1. Cytomegalovirus (CMV) retinitis is the most common ocular opportunistic infection among patients with AIDS. Uncontrolled fulminating disease may give rise to large posterior retinal breaks and retinal detachment. Since the advent of HAART the incidence of CMV retinitis has declined and its rate of progression reduced, even in patients with low CD4+ T-cell counts. It also appears that the rates of second eye involvement and retinal detachment are less than in the pre-HAART era.

2. Retinal artery macroaneurysm is a localized dilatation of a retinal arteriole which usually occurs in the first three orders of the arterial tree. It has a predilection for elderly hypertensive women and involves one eye in 90% of cases. Chronic leakage resulting in retinal oedema with accumulation of hard exudates at the fovea is common and may result in permanent loss of central vision.

3. Diabetes may cause proliferative retinopathy with fibrovascular proliferation along the superotemporal arcade.

4. High myopia is defined as an eye with a refractive error > −6 D and an axial length of the globe >26 mm. It affects approximately 0.5% of the general population and 30% of myopic eyes. Degenerative myopia is characterized by progressive and excessive anteroposterior elongation of the globe which is associated with secondary changes involving the sclera, retina, choroid, and optic nerve head. Atrophic maculopathy is the most common cause of visual loss in highly myopic patients.

5. Toxoplasma retinitis is the most common cause of infectious retinitis in immunocompetent individuals. Serous detachment of the macula adjacent to an active focus of activity is a very rare complication.

6. Wet age-related macular degeneration (AMD) is less common but more devastating than dry AMD because it may cause sudden and severe visual loss due to bleeding from CNV.

QUESTION 108

What pathogens are involved?

1. Herpes simplex (HSV) is enveloped with a cuboidal capsule and a linear double-stranded DNA genome. The two subtypes are HSV-1 and HSV-2 which reside equally in almost all ganglia. HSV-1 primarily causes infection above the waist that may affect the face, lips, and eyes, whereas HSV-2 causes venereally acquired infection (genital herpes). Epithelial (dendritic) keratitis is caused by virus replication and is the most common ocular presentation.

2. *Acanthamoeba* spp are ubiquitous free-living protozoa commonly found in soil, fresh or brackish water, and the upper respiratory tract. In developed countries acanthamoeba keratitis is most frequently associated with contact lens wear, especially if tap water is use for cleaning. Perineural corneal infiltrates (radial keratoneuritis) are seen during the first 1–4 weeks and are pathognomonic.

3. *Chlamydia* spp are small, obligate intracellular bacteria that cannot replicate extracellularly and hence depend on host cells. Adult chlamydial (inclusion) conjunctivitis is an oculogenital infection caused by serotypes D–K of *C. trachomatis*. Transmission is by autoinoculation from genital secretions although eye-to-eye spread may account for about 10% of cases. Ocular involvement is characterized by follicular conjunctivitis and tender preauricular

lymphadenopathy. Peripheral corneal infiltrates may appear 2–3 weeks after the onset of conjunctivitis.

4. Infectious crystalline keratitis is a rare, indolent infection usually associated with long-term topical steroid therapy most frequently following penetrating keratoplasty. It is characterized by slowly progressive, grey-white, branching opacities in the anterior or mid stroma with minimal inflammation and usually intact overlying epithelium. **Strep. viridans** is most commonly isolated although numerous other bacteria and fungi have been implicated.

5. Trachoma is chronic conjunctival inflammation caused by infection with serotypes A, B, Ba, and C of **C. trachomatis**. Initial infection is self-limiting and resolves without scarring but repeated infection can lead to corneal opacification.

6. Fungi are micro-organisms that have rigid walls and multiple chromosomes containing both DNA and RNA. The main types are filamentous (e.g. **Aspergillus** spp) and yeasts (**Candida** spp). Risk factors for keratitis are trauma, particularly with vegetable matter, chronic ocular surface disease, and epithelial defects, diabetes, systemic immunosuppression, and hydrophilic contact lenses. Keratitis is characterized by grey-yellow stromal infiltrates with indistinct margins, often surrounded by satellite lesions.

QUESTION 109

What treatment has been performed and for what reason?

1. Nd:YAG laser iridotomy to create an artificial pupil in congenital ectopia lentis et pupil-

lae which is a rare AR, bilateral condition characterized by displacement of the pupils and lens in opposite directions. The pupils are small and difficult to dilate.

2. Nd:YAG laser capsulotomy for posterior capsular opacification is indicated for diminished visual acuity, or the presence of diplopia or glare due to capsular wrinkling.

3. Nd:YAG laser peripheral iridotomy for pupil-block angle closure. Primary angle closure occurs in anatomically predisposed eyes in which elevation of IOP occurs as a consequence of obstruction of aqueous outflow by occlusion of the trabecular meshwork by the peripheral iris. The condition is an ophthalmic emergency. Peripheral laser iridotomy is aimed at re-establishing communication between the posterior and anterior chambers by making an opening in the peripheral iris. It is important to confirm that the angle is open after peripheral iridotomy even if the IOP is normal.

4. Brachytherapy of a choroidal melanoma has caused surrounding atrophy of the RPE and choroid.

5. Grid argon laser photocoagulation for diffuse diabetic maculopathy in which light intensity burns are applied to areas of diffuse retinal thickening more than 500 μm from the centre of the macula and 500 μm from the temporal edge of the disc.

6. Laser photocoagulation for retinopathy of prematurity of avascular immature retina is indicated in infants with threshold disease to prevent retinal detachment. This is successful in 85% of cases.

What are these complications of trabeculectomy?

1. Cataract due to shallow anterior chamber. Severe and sustained shallowing is uncommon, because the chamber re-forms spontaneously in most cases. However, those that do not may develop severe complications such as peripheral anterior synechiae, corneal endothelial damage, and cataract.

2. Blebitis. Glaucoma filtration-associated infection is classified as limited to the bleb (blebitis) or endophthalmitis, although there is some overlap. The incidence of blebitis following trabeculectomy with mitomycin is estimated to be 5% per year and endophthalmitis about 1% per year. Blebitis is characterized by a white bleb that contains inflammatory material but anterior uveitis is absent, and the red reflex normal.

3. Bleb leakage of aqueous is characterized by a positive Seidel test in which aqueous dilutes the fluorescein-stained tear film.

4. Encapsulated bleb (Tenon cyst) typically develops 2–8 weeks postoperatively and is associated with failure of filtration. It is characterized by a localized, highly elevated, dome-shaped, fluid-filled cavity of hypertrophied Tenon capsule with engorged surface blood vessels.

5. Ciliochoroidal detachment may develop in eyes with persistent low intraocular pressures, usually as a result of overfiltration. In severe cases it is possible to visualize the extreme fundus periphery on the slit-lamp without the use of a contact lens.

6. Hypotonous maculopathy is caused by very low intraocular pressure (usually <6 mmHg) particularly when adjunctive antimetabolites are used. It is characterized by chorioretinal folds that tend to radiate outwards in a branching fashion from the optic disc often associated with disc oedema. Delayed normalization of intraocular pressure may result in permanent macular changes and poor vision.

QUESTION 111

Match the skin (1–3) with the eye (A–C)

I and A

Reiter syndrome is characterized by the triad of non-specific (non-gonococcal) urethritis, conjunctivitis, and arthritis. About 85% of patients are positive for HLA-B27 but the diagnosis is clinical and is based on the presence of arthritis and other characteristic manifestation such as **keratoderma blenorrhagica** (**1**). **Conjunctivitis** is very common and usually follows the urethritis by about 2 weeks and precedes the arthritis. The inflammation is usually mild, bilateral, and mucopurulent with a papillary (**A**) or follicular reaction. Spontaneous resolution occurs within 7–10 days and treatment is not required. Other ocular manifestations are acute anterior uveitis, and rarely, nummular keratitis, episcleritis, scleritis, papillitis, and retinal vasculitis.

2 and C

Rheumatoid arthritis (RA) is an autoimmune systemic disease characterized by a symmetrical, destructive, deforming, inflammatory polyarthropathy, in association with a spectrum of extra-articular manifestations and circulating antiglobulin antibodies. Subcutaneous **'rheumatoid' nodules** over prominences are common (**2**). **Scleromalacia perforans** is a specific type of necrotizing scleritis without inflammation that typically affects elderly women with long-standing RA. It is characterized by painless, very slowly progressive scleral thinning and exposure of the underlying uvea (**C**). Other ocular manifestations of RA are keratoconjunctivitis sicca, inflammatory scleritis, peripheral keratitis, and rarely, acquired superior oblique tendon sheath syndrome.

3 and B

Atopic eczema (dermatitis) is an idiopathic, often familial, skin condition, which may be associated with asthma and hay fever. **Flexural eczema** is characterized by symmetrical involvement of elbow and knee flexures, wrists (**3**), and ankles by dry, lichenified or excoriated skin. **Atopic keratoconjunctivitis**, which may result in persistent corneal epithelial defects and peripheral vascularization (**B**), develops in a minority of patients. Other ocular manifestations include madarosis, staphylococcal blepharitis, keratoconus, early-onset cataract, and rarely, retinal detachment.

QUESTION 112

Diabetic retinopathy – is treatment required?

1. No. Mild background diabetic retinopathy (DR) with small exudates and vascular lesions does not require treatment because the risk of severe visual loss is very small.

2. Yes. Severe proliferative DR with extensive disc neovascularization requires panretinal laser photocoagulation because the risk of severe visual loss within two years is high.

3. No. End-stage background DR with a large plaque at the macula does not require treatment because visual loss is irreversible.

4. Maybe. Premacular subhyaloid haemorrhage, if dense and persistent, may be considered for vitrectomy because, if untreated, the internal limiting membrane or posterior hyaloid face may serve as a scaffold for subsequent fibrovascular proliferation and consequent tractional macular detachment or macular epiretinal membrane formation.

5. Occasionally. Pre-proliferative DR is characterized by venous changes and deep haemorrhages. Patients should be watched closely because of the high risk of developing proliferative DR. Laser treatment is usually not appropriate unless regular follow-up is not possible, or vision in the fellow eye has been already lost due to proliferative disease.

6. No. Retinal fibrosis in the absence of neovascularization does not require treatment because photocoagulation only influences the vascular component. However, the patient should be watched because there is still a risk of tractional retinal detachment.

QUESTION 113

Match the orbital lesion (1–3) with the CT (A–C)

I and C

Lacrimal gland carcinoma has caused proptosis, inferior globe displacement, periorbital oedema, and epibulbar congestion due to extension to involve the superior orbital fissure (**1**). **Coronal CT** shows a mass with spotty calcification in the lacrimal fossa, and contiguous erosion of bone (**C**). Lacrimal gland carcinomas are rare tumours which carry a high morbidity and mortality. Presentation is in the fourth to fifth decades with a history shorter than that of a benign tumour. Pain is a frequent feature of malignancy but may also occur with inflammatory lesions.

2 and A

Orbital cellulitis has caused proptosis, periorbital oedema, and mechanical ptosis (**2**). **Axial CT** shows preseptal and orbital opacification (**A**). Bacterial orbital cellulitis is a life-threatening infection of the soft tissues behind the orbital septum. It can occur at any age but is more common in children. Important features include malaise, ophthalmoplegia, and optic nerve dysfunction.

3 and B

Optic nerve glioma has caused severe non-congestive, non-axial proptosis (**3**). **Axial CT** shows fusiform optic nerve enlargement (**B**). Optic nerve glioma is a slow-growing, pilocytic astrocytoma which typically affects children, girls more often than boys. Approximately 30% of patients have associated neurofibromatosis-1.

QUESTION 114

What are these uncommon fundus conditions?

1. Double branch vein occlusion involving both the superior and inferior temporal branches.

2. Progressive bifocal chorioretinal atrophy is an AD condition characterized by a focus of chorioretinal atrophy temporal to the disc which extends in all directions. A similar lesion develops nasally and the end result manifests two separate areas of chorioretinal atrophy separated by a normal segment.

3. Sclerochoroidal calcification (ossification) is characterized by multiple, yellow placoid lesions typically located along vascular arcades.

4. Congenital arteriovenous communication is usually asymptomatic although occasionally it may leak or become occluded.

5. Subretinal cysticercus cyst with retinal detachment. The larvae enter the subretinal space and can pass into the vitreous where released toxins incite an intense inflammatory reaction which may ultimately lead to severe visual loss.

6. Opaque (myelinated) nerve fibres are characterized by feathery streaks running within the retinal nerve fibre layer towards the disc. Patients with extensive involvement may be highly myopic, anisometropic, and amblyopic.

QUESTION 115

What are these ocular motility defects?

1. Bilateral inferior oblique overaction. The eyes are straight in the primary position (**A**); overaction of the left inferior oblique on right gaze (**B**); overaction of the right inferior oblique on left gaze (**C**). Inferior oblique overaction is common in early-onset esotropia, and may also be secondary to superior oblique underaction.

2. Dissociated vertical deviation (DVD) is characterized by straight eyes in the primary position (**A**); up-drift of the left eye under cover (**B**); up-drift of the right eye under cover and down-drift of the left eye (**C**). DVD may appear several years after initial surgery for early-onset esotropia. Surgical correction is indicated when it is cosmetically unacceptable.

QUESTION 116

What are these subtle signs?

1. Herbert pits are shallow superior limbal depressions that develop following resolution of conjunctival follicles in trachoma.

2. Posterior polymorphous dystrophy is a rare, innocuous, and asymptomatic condition in which corneal endothelial cells display characteristics similar to epithelium. It is characterized by subtle band-like, vesicular or diffuse opacities which may be asymmetrical.

3. Glaucomflecken are small, grey-white, anterior subcapsular or capsular opacities in the pupillary zone that are diagnostic of a previous attack of congestive angle closure.

4. Meesman dystrophy is a very rare innocuous AD condition. It is characterized by myriads of tiny intraepithelial cysts of uniform size but variable density maximal centrally that extend towards but do not reach the limbus.

5. Pseudoexfoliation (PXE) on the pupillary margin associated with pupillary ruff defects.

6. Congenital pigment deposits on the anterior lens capsule.

QUESTION 117

What treatment is being performed?

1. Probing of the nasolacrimal ducts is indicated in infants with delayed canalization that has not resolved spontaneously by the age of 12–18 months.

2. Diode laser cycloablation lowers intraocular pressure by partly destroying the ciliary secretory epithelium, thereby reducing aqueous secretion. It is used mainly in glaucomatous eyes in which conventional drainage surgery has little or no chance of success.

3. Cryoablation of lashes is indicated for severe trichiasis and distichiasis. Complications include skin necrosis, depigmentation, damage to meibomian glands, and shallow notching of the lid margin.

4. Reconstruction of the anterior lamella of the eyelid with a free skin graft is performed following extensive excision of the lower lid, usually in the treatment of malignant tumours. Reconstruction of the posterior lamella may involve grafting of hard palate, tarsus, buccal mucous membrane, or a Hughes graft from the upper lid.

5. Pars plana vitrectomy is indicated in the treatment of complicated rhegmatogenous retinal detachments such as those associated with proliferative vitreoretinopathy or giant tears. It is also indicated in eyes with tractional retinal detachments, and non-resolving vitreous opacities.

6. Photocoagulation prior to endoresection of choroidal melanoma is performed to prevent retinal detachment after the tumour has been resected.

QUESTION 118

What multiple signs do these patients show?

1. Albinism and **herpes simplex rash**.

2. Small right phthisical eye and a **large left globe** due to very high myopia.

3. Right lid retraction and **left ptosis** in myasthenia gravis.

4. Right herpes zoster ophthalmicus and **facial palsy.**

5. Long-standing acne rosacea and a **red right eye and thickened upper lid** probably due to recurrent chalazion formation.

6. Bilateral naevus flammeus, hypertrophy of the upper lips and **right buphthalmos** in Sturge–Weber syndrome.

QUESTION 119

Match the corneal dystrophy (1–3) with the stain (A–C)

1 and A

Reis–Bückler is an AD condition which presents in the first to second decades with painful recurrent corneal erosions. It is characterized by grey-white, round, and polygonal opacities in Bowman layer, most dense centrally (**1**). Corneal sensation is reduced and visual impairment may occur due to scarring at Bowman layer. **Histology** shows replacement of Bowman layer and the epithelial basement membrane with fibrous tissue (**A**).

2 and C

Lattice dystrophy is an AD condition that presents at the end of the first decade with recurrent erosions which may precede typical stromal changes. It is characterized by stromal lattice lines that spare the periphery. Later a generalized stromal haze progressively impairs vision and may obscure the lattice lines (**2**). **Histology** shows amyloid that stains with Congo red (**C**).

3 and B

Macular dystrophy is an AR condition that presents in the first decade with gradual visual deterioration. It is characterized by a central anterior stromal haze associated with greyish-white, dense, focal, poorly delineated spots in the anterior stroma centrally and posterior stroma in the periphery (**3**). **Histology** shows abnormally close packing of collagen in the corneal lamellae and abnormal aggregations of glycosaminoglycans which stain with Prussian blue and colloidal iron (**B**).

QUESTION 120

Which is the odd one out?

2 Posterior synechiae

These do not occur in Fuchs uveitis syndrome (FUS).

Cataract (**1**) is very common and often the presenting feature of FUS; **secondary glaucoma** occurs in long-standing cases and may give rise to disc damage (**3**); **keratic precipitates** are characteristically small, round or stellate, grey-white in colour, distributed throughout the endothelium, and may be associated with feathery fibrin filaments (**4**); gonioscopy may show twig-like vessels in the angle (**5**) that bleed on anterior chamber paracentesis; **vitritis** and stringy opacities are common and may be dense (**6**).

QUESTION 121

What urinary abnormalities may be present?

1. Increased ornithine in **gyrate atrophy**, which is an AR condition in which deficiency of ornithine aminotransferase leads to elevated ornithine levels in the plasma, urine, CSF, and aqueous humour. The fundus shows patches of chorioretinal atrophy and vitreous degeneration.

2. Increased vanillyl mandelic acid due to catecholamine secretion by **neuroblastoma** which is one of the most common childhood malignancies. It arises from primitive neuroblasts of the sympathetic chain, most commonly in the abdomen, followed by the thorax and pelvis. Orbital metastases present with an abrupt onset of proptosis accompanied by a superior orbital mass and lid ecchymosis.

3. Glycosuria in **diabetes mellitus.** The fundus shows extensive venous dilatation and beading, the hallmark of pre-proliferative disease.

4. Homocysteine in **homocystinuria.** The latter is an AR disorder of methionine metabolism caused by deficiency of cystathionine-beta-synthetase leading to accumulation of methionine and homocysteine. Patients have blond hair, a malar flush, a marfanoid habitus, and a tendency to thromboses. Progressive ectopia lentis, associated with disintegrated zonules, is present in 90% of patients. The lens dislocates inferiorly or into the anterior chamber.

5. Haematuria in **Alport syndrome**, which is a rare XLD abnormality of glomerular basement membrane, often associated with sensorineural deafness. Presentation is frequently with haematuria followed by chronic renal failure. Strong ocular associations are anterior lenticonus, which causes a characteristic abnormality of the red reflex, and macular flecks.

6. Increased homogentistic acid in **alkaptonuria,** which is an AR aminoacidopathy due to a deficiency of homogentistic acid oxidase. This results in accumulation of homogentistic acid in collagenous tissue such as cartilage, tendon, and sclera (ochronosis).

QUESTION 122

Which systemic drugs may cause these problems?

1. Chlorpromazine (Largactil) is used as a sedative and to treat psychotic illnesses. Some patients on long-term therapy develop innocuous, fine, stellate granules on the anterior lens capsule within the pupillary area. Other toxic effects are endothelial deposits, and rarely, mild retinopathy.

2. Tetracyclines are broad-spectrum antibiotics which are used in ophthalmology mainly to treat chlamydial infections, acne rosacea, and Lyme disease. The drugs are deposited in growing bone and teeth (being bound to calcium) causing staining and occasionally dental hypoplasia. They should therefore not be administered to children under 12 years or pregnant or breast-feeding women.

3. Minocycline is a tetracycline with a broader spectrum than the other compounds. Rarely, it may give rise to pigmentation of the skin and conjunctiva, which may be irreversible.

4. Interferon alpha is used in a variety of systemic conditions including Kaposi sarcoma, haemangioma in infancy, high-risk cutaneous melanomas, metastatic renal cell carcinoma, leukaemia, lymphoma, and chronic hepatitis C. Retinopathy characterized by cotton-wool spots and intraretinal haemorrhages may develop, particularly with high-dose therapy.

5. Canthaxanthin is a carotenoid used to enhance sun tanning. If used over prolonged periods of time it may cause the deposition of innocuous, inner retinal, tiny, glistening, yellow deposits, arranged symmetrically in a doughnut shape at the posterior poles.

6. Thioridazine (Melleril) is used to treat schizophrenia and related psychoses. The normal daily dose is 150–600 mg. Doses which exceed 800 mg/day for just a few weeks may be sufficient to cause reduced visual acuity and impairment of dark adaptation. Advanced toxicity gives rise to pigmented plaques associated with diffuse loss of the RPE and choriocapillaris.

QUESTION 123

Match 1 with one of (A–D)

I and C

Molluscum contagiosum is a viral skin infection which typically affects otherwise healthy children with a peak incidence between 2 and 4 years. Transmission is by contact with infected people and then by autoinoculation. A molluscum lesion on the lid margin (**C**) may shed virus into the tear film and give rise to secondary, ipsilateral, chronic, follicular conjunctivitis (**1**).

The other eyelid lesions shown are not associated with conjunctivitis: cyst of Zeis (**A**); discharging external hordeolum (**B**); squamous cell papilloma (**D**).

QUESTION 124

Match the blood film (1–3) with the eye (A–C)

I and C

Chronic lymphocytic leukaemia typically affects elderly patients who manifest hepatosplenomegaly and lymphadenopathy. The course is very long and many patients may die from an unrelated cause. The blood film shows **mature lymphocytosis (1)**. Choroidal infiltration is rare and causes a **leopard skin** appearance (**C**).

2 and B

Sickling haemoglobinopathies are caused by one, or a combination, of abnormal haemoglobins which cause the red blood cell to adopt an anomalous shape under conditions of hypoxia and acidosis. Because these deformed red blood cells are more rigid than healthy cells, they may become impacted in and obstruct small blood vessels. The blood film shows several **sickled cells** and one nucleated red cell in homozygous (HbSS) disease (**2**). **FA** of proliferative retinopathy is characterized by tufts of new vessels ('sea-fans') and extensive peripheral retinal capillary non-perfusion (**B**).

3 and A

Acute myelocytic leukaemia is characterized by replacement of bone marrow by very **immature (blast) cells** (**3**). The disease is most frequently seen in older adults and is curable in 30% of those under the age of 60 years. Anterior segment involvement by leukaemic cells, which is rare, is characterized by iris thickening and **pseudo-hypopyon** (**A**).

QUESTION 125

What do these fluorescein angiograms show?

1. Several choroidal neovascular membranes in **punctate inner choroidopathy**.

2. Extensive hypofluorescence of the posterior fundus due to ischaemia in **acute retinal necrosis**.

3. Choroidal hypofluorescence associated with non-perfusion due to a **choroidal infarct**.

4. Areas of hypofluorescence due to retinal capillary non-perfusion and many areas of hyperfluorescence due to leakage from new vessels in **proliferative diabetic retinopathy**.

5. Hyperfluorescence at the macula due to a window defect and a dark choroid in **Stargardt disease**.

6. Myriads of pin-point areas of hyperfluorescence in **basal laminar drusen**.

QUESTION 126

Hamartoma or choristoma?

Choristomas are benign congenital tumours containing tissue not normally present at that site. Hamartomas are benign congenital tumours containing tissue normally present at that site. Frequently a choristoma or hamartoma may not be clinically apparent at birth and present later in life.

1. Choristoma – solid dermoid presents in early childhood as a smooth, soft, yellowish, subconjunctival mass most frequently located at the infero-temporal limbus. Occasionally the lesions are very large and may virtually encircle the limbus (complex choristoma). Systemic associations include Goldenhar syndrome, and less commonly, Treacher–Collins syndrome and naevus sebaceus of Jadassohn.

2. Hamartoma – capillary haemangioma is the most common tumour of the orbit and periorbital areas in childhood. Girls are affected more commonly than boys. The tumour may present as a small isolated lesion of minimal clinical significance or as a large disfiguring mass that can cause visual impairment. Presentation is usually in the first few weeks of life.

3. Hamartoma – cavernous orbital haemangioma is the most common benign orbital tumour in adults, with a female preponderance of 70%. Although it may develop anywhere in the orbit, it most frequently occurs within the lateral part of the muscle cone just behind the globe. Presentation is in the fourth to fifth decades with slowly progressive unilateral proptosis. The tumour is usually well encapsulated and relatively easy to remove.

4. Hamartoma – retinal astrocytoma is a rare tumour which does not threaten vision. It may occasionally be encountered as an incidental solitary lesion in normal individuals but it is most frequently seen in patients with tuberous sclerosis.

5. Hamartoma – plexiform neurofibroma on the eyelid typically affects patients with neurofibromatosis-1, and causes a characteristic S-shaped deformity.

6. Hamartoma – combined hamartoma of the RPE and retina is a rare, usually unilateral congenital malformation that predominantly affects males. The lesion is composed of RPE, sensory retina, retinal blood vessels, and vitreoretinal membranes. Presentation is in late childhood or early adulthood with strabismus, blurred vision or metamorphopsia.

QUESTION 127

What do these charts show?

1. Left third nerve palsy

• The left chart is much smaller than the right.

• Left exotropia – note that the fixation spots in the inner charts of both eyes are deviated laterally. The deviation is greater on the right chart (when the left eye is fixating), indicating that secondary deviation exceeds the primary – as is typical of paretic squint.
• Left chart shows underaction of all muscles except the lateral rectus.
• Right chart shows overaction of all muscles except the medial rectus and inferior rectus, the 'yokes' of the spared muscles.
• The primary angle of deviation (fixing right eye – FR) in the primary position is −20° and R/L 10°.
• The secondary angle (fixing left eye – FL) is −28° and R/L 12°.

2. Congenital right fourth nerve palsy

• No differences in chart size.
• Primary and secondary deviation R/L 4°.
• Right hypertropia – note that the fixation spot of the right inner chart is deviated upwards and the left is deviated downwards.
• Hypertropia increases on laevoversion and reduces on dextroversion.
• Right chart shows underaction of the superior oblique and overaction of the inferior oblique.
• Left chart shows overaction of the inferior rectus and underaction (inhibitional palsy) of the superior rectus.

QUESTION 128

What do these charts show?

1. Recently acquired right fourth nerve palsy

• Right chart is smaller than the left.
• Right chart shows underaction of the superior oblique and overaction of the inferior oblique.

- Left chart shows overaction of the inferior rectus and underaction (inhibitional palsy) of the superior rectus.
- The primary deviation (FL) is R/L 8°; the secondary deviation FR is R/L17°.

2. Right sixth nerve palsy

- Right chart is smaller than the left.
- Right esotropia – note that the fixation spot of the right inner chart is deviated nasally.
- Right chart shows marked underaction of the lateral rectus and slight overaction of the medial rectus.
- Left chart shows marked overaction of the medial rectus.
- The primary angle FL is +15° and the secondary angle FR +20°.

indicative of previous exposure. A strongly positive result (>15 mm) is usually indicative of active disease (**3**). A negative result usually excludes tuberculosis.

4. En taches de beaugie (candle wax drippings) describes perivenous exudates that are indicative of severe periphlebitis in sarcoidosis.

5. Fleurettes (small flowers) is a histological description of retinoblastoma in which clusters of cells with long cytoplasmic processes project through a fenestrated membrane resembling a bouquet of flowers.

6. Peau d'orange (orange skin) consists of mottled pigmentation in eyes with angioid streaks.

QUESTION 129

What have these conditions in common?

They are all French descriptions

1. Iris bombé describes anterior bowing of the iris due to pupil block that prevents passage of aqueous from the posterior chamber to the anterior chamber. Iris bombé is most often caused by seclusion pupillae (i.e. 360° posterior synechiae).

2. Café au lait (coffee with milk) spots are light-brown macules most commonly found on the trunk in patients with neurofibromatosis-1. They appear during the first year of life and increase in size and number throughout childhood.

3. Mantoux test involves the intradermal injection of purified protein derivative of *M. tuberculosis*. A positive result is characterized by the development of an induration of 5–14 mm within 48 hours, and is

QUESTION 130

Which of these conditions require treatment with antibiotics?

1. Simple episcleritis does **not require** antibiotic treatment. If the patient is seen within 48 hours of onset of the first attack, topical steroids may be used half hourly during the day for two days, then q.i.d. for one day, b.d. for one day and daily for two days. Treatment of extremely frequent or disabling attacks involves a systemic non-steroidal anti-inflammatory drug (NSAID) such as flurbiprofen 100 mg t.i.d. for 10 days. If recurrences occur thereafter, long-term treatment or a change of drug may be necessary.

2. Bacterial keratitis has the potential to progress rapidly to corneal perforation and therefore **requires urgent** antibiotic therapy. Even small axial lesions can cause surface irregularity and scarring that can lead to significant loss of vision. Topical broad spectrum antibiotics (fluoroquinolones) are initially instilled at hourly intervals day and night for 24–48 hours. The frequency can be reduced to 2-hourly during waking hours for a further 48 hours, and then q.i.d. until the epithelium has healed.

3. Papillary conjunctivitis with giant papillae does **not require** antibiotics because it occurs in allergic conditions such as reaction to contact lens wear, vernal disease, and atopic keratoconjunctivitis. According to the underlying cause and severity treatment involves topical and occasionally a systemic NSAID, as well as topical steroids.

4. Orbital cellulitis is a life-threatening condition which **requires** very urgent treatment with intramuscular ceftazidime 1 g every 8 hours, and oral metronidazole 500 mg to cover anaerobes. Treatment should be continued until the patient is apyrexial for 4 days.

5. Acute allergic oedema is caused by insect bites, angioedema or urticaria and does **not require** antibiotics. Spontaneous resolution is the rule although in severe cases systemic antihistamines may be helpful.

6. Chronic contact dermatitis is caused by exposure to a medication, a preservative or a cosmetic and does **not require** antibiotics. The mainstay of treatment is stopping exposure to the allergen.

QUESTION 131

What are the HLA associations of these inflammatory conditions?

1. Behçet disease is an idiopathic, multisystem disease characterized by recurrent episodes of orogenital ulceration and vasculitis which may involve small, medium, and large veins and arteries. The disease typically affects patients from the eastern Mediterranean region and Japan and is strongly associated with **HLA-B51** in different ethnic groups. However, it is not clear whether the HLA-B51 itself is the pathogenic gene or some other gene is in linkage disequilibrium with HLA-B51. During the acute stage of the systemic disease the fundus may show white, necrotic infiltrates which heal without scarring.

2. Acute anterior uveitis with a fibrinous exudate is strongly associated with **HLA-B27**. The prevalence is 50% in patients with no underlying systemic disease, and 90% with an associated spondyloarthropathy such as ankylosing spondylitis and Reiter syndrome. The anterior uveitis associated with HLA-B27 is typically severe, recurrent, and with a tendency to the formation of posterior synechiae. Patients with acute anterior uveitis, who do not carry HLA-B27, tend to have a more benign course with fewer recurrences.

3. Vogt–Koyanagi–Harada (V–K–H) syndrome is an idiopathic, multisystem, autoimmune disease against melanocytes causing inflammation of melanocyte-containing tissues such as the uvea, ear, and meninges. V–K–H predominantly affects Hispanics, Japanese, and pigmented individuals. In different racial groups the disease is associated with **HLA-DR1** and **HLA-DR4**, suggesting a common immunogenic predisposition. In practice, V–K–H can be subdivided into Vogt–Koyanagi disease, characterized mainly by skin changes and anterior uveitis, and Harada disease in which posterior segment disease predominates. The acute phase is characterized by multifocal detachments of the sensory retina, followed by exudative retinal detachment.

4. Acute posterior multifocal placoid pigment epitheliopathy (APMPPE) is an uncommon, idiopathic, usually bilateral condition, which typically affects individuals in the third to sixth decades. It affects both sexes equally and is associated with **HLA-B7** and **HLA-DR2**. In about one-third of patients APMPPE follows a flu-like illness and occasionally it may be the initial manifestation of a CNS angiitis. The acute stage is characterized by multiple, large, placoid lesions which typically start at the posterior pole and then extend to the post-equatorial fundus.

5. Serpiginous choroidopathy is an uncommon, chronic, recurrent disease which is usually bilateral but the extent of involvement is frequently asymmetrical. It affects individuals in the fourth to sixth decades of life, men more than women, and is associated with **HLA-B7**. The disease has a chronic, recurrent evolution, and may remain inactive for months or years. Active lesions are grey-white or yellow. They develop first around the optic disc and then gradually spread towards the macula and periphery.

6. Birdshot retinochoroidopathy is an uncommon, idiopathic, chronic, recurrent, bilateral disease which typically affects individuals in the fifth to seventh decades of life, predominantly females. Over 95% of patients are positive for **HLA-A29**. Active lesions are small, ill-defined, cream-coloured spots in the posterior pole and mid-periphery.

QUESTION 132

What are these ocular motility defects?

1. Right Brown syndrome characterized by straight eyes in the primary position (**A**); limited right elevation in adduction (**B**); absence of superior oblique overaction (**C**). The condition is usually congenital and rarely acquired.

2. Bilateral internuclear ophthalmoplegia characterized by limited right adduction on left gaze

(**A**); limited left adduction on right gaze (**B**); absence of convergence (**C**) when the lesion is extensive. Important causes include demyelination, vascular disease, brainstem tumours, and trauma.

QUESTION 133

What are these subtle fundus lesions?

1. Hollenhorst plaque at the bifurcation of the inferotemporal artery. The plaque is composed of cholesterol derived from an atheromatous plaque at the carotid bifurcation, or less commonly, the aortic arch. It rarely causes significant obstruction and is often asymptomatic.

2. Multiple evanescent white dot syndrome (MEWDS) is an uncommon, idiopathic, usually unilateral, self-limiting disease which typically affects individuals between the ages of 20–40 years, particularly females. It presents with sudden onset of decreased vision or paracentral scotomas which may be associated with photopsia, typically affecting the temporal visual field. The fundus shows numerous, very small, ill-defined, white dots at the level of the outer retina and inner choroid involving the posterior pole and mid-periphery but sparing the macula.

3. Retinal tear in flat retina.

4. Very early retinal haemangioblastoma characterized by a small, well-defined red lesion associated with a slightly dilated feeding artery and draining vein.

5. Familial internal limiting membrane dystrophy is a rare AD condition that presents in the third to fourth decades with visual loss. The posterior pole manifests a glistening inner retinal surface.

Prognosis is poor with visual loss occurring by the sixth decade due to retinoschisis, retinal oedema, and retinal folds.

6. Adult-onset foveomacular vitelliform dystrophy presents in the fourth to sixth decades with mild to moderate decrease of visual acuity and sometimes metamorphopsia, although often the condition is discovered by chance. It is characterized by bilateral, symmetrical, round or oval, slightly elevated, yellowish subfoveal deposits, about one-third of a disc diameter in size, often centered by a pigmented spot. Prognosis is good in the majority of cases.

QUESTION 134

At what age do these conditions present?

1. Anterior ischaemic optic neuropathy typically presents in the **eighth decade** with acute onset of unilateral visual loss. Ophthalmoscopy shows a pale swollen optic nerve head with peripapillary splinter-shaped haemorrhages. Giant cell arteritis is an important cause which should be excluded as systemic steroid therapy usually prevents involvement of the second eye.

2. Granular dystrophy type 2 (Avellino) presents in the **second decade**. It is characterized by fine superficial opacities consisting of rings, discs or snowflakes, most dense centrally (resembling those seen in granular dystrophy type 1), with associated deeper linear opacities reminiscent of lattice dystrophy.

3. Embryonic sarcoma presents in the **first decade** (average age 7 years) with rapidly progressive proptosis which may initially mimic an inflammatory process. MR shows a poorly defined mass of homogeneous density.

4. Retinoblastoma presents within the **first year** of life in bilateral cases and around the age of **2 years** if the tumour is unilateral.

5. Choroidal melanoma typically affects patients in the **seventh decade** of life.

6. Persistent anterior fetal vasculature presents at **birth** with unilateral leukocoria in a microphthalmic eye. It is characterized by a retrolental mass into which elongated ciliary processes are inserted.

QUESTION 135

What treatment has been performed?

1. Exenteration with removal of part of the lateral orbital wall. The procedure involves removal of the globe and intraorbital contents, which can be performed with or without preservation of the eyelids. It is indicated for advanced malignancies such as orbital extension of intraocular melanoma, embryonal sarcoma, and lacrimal gland carcinoma, which may also require removal of adjacent bone, as in this case.

2. Trabeculectomy. The eye also shows congenital ectropion uveae which may be associated with developmental glaucoma, particularly in patients with neurofibromatosis-1.

3. Scleral grafting may be required in eyes with severe thinning with impending perforation, usually secondary to necrotizing scleritis. Attempts should be made to preserve as much healthy conjunctiva surrounding the necrotic scleral bed as possible to reduce the size of the postoperative epithelial defect overlying the graft.

4. Glaucoma drainage shunts are plastic devices which create a communication between the anterior chamber and sub-Tenon space. Indications include uncontrolled glaucoma despite previous trabeculectomy with adjunctive antimetabolites, secondary glaucomas where routine trabeculectomy even with adjunctive antimetabolites is unlikely to succeed, and eyes with severe conjunctival scarring.

5. Scleral rings, consisting of a large haptic contact lens with the central zone removed, are occasionally used to prevent symblepharon formation in eyes with severe cicatrizing conjunctivitis, such as in ocular cicatricial pemphigoid and Stevens–Johnson syndrome.

6. Intravitreal steroid injections consisting of triamcinolone acetonide are used to treat intractable chronic macular oedema associated with diabetes, retinal vein occlusion, pseudophakia, uveitis, and radiation retinopathy. It has also been used to treat choroidal neovascularization associated with wet age-related macular degeneration, presumed ocular histoplasmosis syndrome, and choroiditis.

QUESTION 136

What have these conditions in common?

They are all associated with 'pseudo'

1. Pseudopterygium is overgrowth of bulbar conjunctiva onto the cornea, most often in association with Terrien marginal degeneration, peripheral corneal ulceration, or chemical burns. The lesion is fixed only at its apex to the cornea, in contrast to a true pterygium which is adherent to underlying structures throughout and only develops medially.

2. Pseudohypopyon describes stage 3 juvenile Best macular dystrophy which may occur at puberty in which the superior part of the lesion becomes absorbed but the inferior portion persists.

3. Pseudogerontoxon may develop in patients with recurrent limbitis associated with vernal keratoconjunctivitis. It resembles a local area of corneal arcus adjacent to a previously inflamed segment of the limbus.

4. Pseudoexfoliation refers to the deposition of a grey-white, fibrillogranular material in the anterior segment, which may lead to raised intraocular pressure as a result of trabecular blockage. Deposits on the anterior lens capsule are characteristic.

5. Pseudoesotropia is the false impression of convergent squint in children with prominent epicanthic folds, or a short inter-pupillary distance.

6. Pseudoxanthoma elasticum is a rare disorder characterized by progressive calcification, fragmentation, and degeneration of elastic fibres in the skin, eye, and cardiovascular system. The skin acquires a 'plucked chicken' appearance and then becomes progressively loose, thin, and delicate. Fifty per cent of patients with angioid streaks have co-existent pseudoxanthoma elasticum (Groenblad–Strandberg syndrome).

QUESTION 137

What are the systemic associations of these conditions?

1. Acute iritis primarily occurs in patients who suffer from a spondyloarthropathy (ankylosing spondylitis, Reiter syndrome, and psoriatic arthritis) and are carriers of HLA-B27. Other important associations include acute-onset sarcoidosis, Behçet disease, and syphilis. Uncommon associations include inflammatory bowel disease (ulcerative colitis, Crohn disease), nephritis (tubulointerstitial nephritis, IgA glomerulonephritis), and relapsing polychondritis.

2. Keratoconjunctivitis sicca occurs in primary Sjögren syndrome, and in secondary Sjögren syndrome which may be associated with a wide variety of diseases, most notably: rheumatoid arthritis, systemic lupus erythematosus, scleroderma, dermatomyositis, polymyositis, mixed connective tissue disease, relapsing polychondritis, and primary biliary cirrhosis.

3. Peripheral corneal ulceration may occur in rheumatoid arthritis, Wegener granulomatosis, polyarteritis nodosa, systemic lupus erythematosus, and relapsing polychondritis.

4. Granulomatous uveitis occurs in chronic sarcoidosis, sympathetic ophthalmitis, Vogt–Koyanagi–Harada syndrome, toxoplasmosis, syphilis, and late-onset postoperative endophthalmitis. Some authorities also consider Fuchs uveitis syndrome to be granulomatous because of the presence of Koeppe nodules, despite the fact that mutton-fat keratic precipitates are absent.

5. Conjunctivitis may be associated with atopic dermatitis, Reiter syndrome, Stevens–Johnson syndrome, cicatricial pemphigoid, chlamydial genital infection, and Kawasaki disease.

6. Necrotizing scleritis occurs in rheumatoid arthritis, Wegener granulomatosis, relapsing polychondritis, polyarteritis nodosa, and systemic lupus erythematosus. Uncommon associations include spondyloarthropathies, Behçet disease, sarcoidosis, and gout.

QUESTION 138

Match the eye (1–3) with the histology (A–C)

1 and C

Embryonal sarcoma ('rhabdomyosarcoma') is the most common primary orbital malignancy of childhood. The tumour is derived from undifferentiated mesenchymal cell rests, which have the potential to differentiate into striated muscle. Presentation is in the first decade (average 7 years) with rapidly progressive unilateral proptosis which may mimic an inflammatory process (**1**). Histology of differentiated tumours show elongated and strap-like cells with a 'tadpole' or 'tennis-racket' configuration with (**C**) or without cross-striations.

2 and B

Choroidal melanoma (**2**) is the most common intraocular malignancy in adults and accounts for 90% of all uveal melanomas. The two main histological types are spindle cell and mixed. The latter is composed of a mixture of spindle and epithelioid cells. Spindle cell tumours are characterized by tightly arranged fusiform cells with indistinct membranes and slender or plump oval nuclei (**B**). A tumour with a preponderance of epithelioid cells carries an unfavourable prognosis.

3 and A

Lacrimal gland mixed cell tumour (pleomorphic adenoma) arising from the palpebral lobe of the lacrimal gland may be visible on everting the eyelid (**3**). Histology shows glandular tissue, and squamous differentiation with keratin formation (**A**).

QUESTION 139

Match the fundus (1–3) with the gonioscopy (A–C)

1 and A

Sympathetic ophthalmitis is a bilateral granulomatous panuveitis occurring after penetrating trauma, often associated with uveal prolapse or less frequently, following intraocular surgery – usually multiple vitreoretinal procedures. The traumatized eye is referred to as the *exciting* eye and the fellow eye, which also develops uveitis, is the *sympathizing* eye. The fundus shows multifocal choroidal infiltrates in the mid-periphery (**1**), and inflammatory nodules may be seen on gonioscopy (**A**).

2 and B

Severe blunt ocular trauma may cause choroidal rupture and subretinal haemorrhage (**2**). Weeks to months later, a white crescent-shaped, streak of exposed underlying sclera concentric with the optic disc becomes visible. Gonioscopy may also show angle recession (**B**) consisting of a tear extending into the face of the ciliary body which later may be associated with elevation of intraocular pressure.

3 and C

Ischaemic central retinal vein occlusion is characterized by rapid onset venous obstruction resulting in decreased retinal perfusion, capillary closure, and retinal hypoxia. Fundoscopy shows severe tortuosity and engorgement of all branches of the central retinal vein, and extensive dot-blot and flame-shaped haemorrhages involving the peripheral retina and posterior pole (**3**). Rubeosis iridis develops in about 50% of eyes, usually between 2 and 4 months (100-day glaucoma), and unless vigorous panretinal photocoagulation is performed

there is a high risk of neovascular glaucoma due to angle closure (**C**).

QUESTION 140

What is the gender preponderance of these conditions?

1. Pigment dispersion syndrome is characterized by trabecular hyperpigmentation which may be associated with elevation of intraocular pressure. The condition typically affects young **males** who are also frequently myopic.

2. Thyrotoxicosis typically affects **females**. Histology of extraocular muscle and orbit in thyroid eye disease shows infiltration with lymphocytes and plasma cells.

3. Age-related macular hole typically affects elderly **females**. OCT of stage 3 hole shows a full-thickness defect more than 400 µm in diameter with an attached posterior hyaloid face, with or without a pseudo-operculum.

4. Coats disease has a predilection for young **males**. It is an idiopathic retinal telangiectasis characterized by intraretinal and subretinal exudation. FA is useful in delineating the vascular anomalies.

5. Retinal artery macroaneurysm typically affects hypertensive elderly **females**. It is characterized by a localized dilatation of a retinal arteriole that may rupture or leak. Spontaneous involution is, however, common and may precede or follow leakage or haemorrhage. FA shows partial hyperfluorescence of the lesion and associated hypofluorescence due to blockage by blood.

6. Choroideremia is a rare XLR disorder affecting only **males**. It is characterized by progressive, diffuse degeneration of the choroid, RPE, and retinal photo-receptors that presents in the first decade with nyctalopia. FA shows filling of the retinal vessels and progressive non-perfusion of the choroidal vessels, and choriocapillaris.

QUESTION 141

What is this disease?

Acquired immunodeficiency syndrome (AIDS) is caused by the human immunodeficiency virus (HIV). Important manifestations include severe herpes zoster ophthalmicus (**1**), monilial infection of the mouth and tongue (**2**), Kaposi sarcoma (**3**), *Pneumocystis carinii* pneumonia (**4**), HIV wasting syndrome (**5**), and intracranial lymphoma (**6**). The progression of HIV infection is as follows: an acute seroconversion illness, an asymptomatic phase, and symptomatic disease characterized by opportunistic infections, tumours, and other manifestations.

QUESTION 142

At what level is the haemorrhage?

1. Retinal nerve fibre layer haemorrhages arise from superficial precapillary arterioles and because of the arrangement of the retinal nerve fibre layer they are flame-shaped. They are found at the posterior pole or in relation to the optic disc, but seldom in the peripheral retina. Important causes include retinal venous occlusion, diabetes, hypertension, and papilloedema.

2. Deep intraretinal haemorrhages arise from the venous end of capillaries and are located in the compact middle layers of the retina with a resultant 'dot' and 'blot' configuration. 'Dot' haemorrhages are small, round, and of uniform density. 'Blot' haemorrhages occupy the entire thickness of the retina and are larger and darker. In the peripheral retina, the retinal nerve fibre layer is thin, so most retinal haemorrhages assume a dot and blot configuration. Large blotchy haemorrhages are indicative of retinal ischaemia and are an important feature of pre-proliferative diabetic retinopathy.

3. Vitreous haemorrhage is caused either by bleeding from neovascular tissue, as in proliferative diabetic retinopathy, or breakthrough of a large subretinal haemorrhage.

4. Subretinal haemorrhage is located between the photoreceptors and the RPE. The haemorrhage is usually large, bright red and has an indistinct margin. Important causes include blunt ocular trauma, choroidal neovascularization, and ruptured retinal artery macroaneurysm.

5. Sub-RPE haemorrhage is derived from the choroid and enters the space between the RPE and Bruch membrane. The haemorrhage is dark red and extensive with a more distinct border than a subretinal bleed. Choroidal neovascularization is by far the most common cause (haemorrhagic detachment of the RPE).

6. Subhyaloid (preretinal) haemorrhage is located between the posterior vitreous face and the internal limiting membrane. It is bright red, usually solitary, and located at the posterior pole. Initially the lesion is round although later it may settle with gravity and assume a boat-shaped configuration.

QUESTION 143

What multiple signs are present?

1. Bilateral proptosis and **lid retraction** and a **thyroidectomy scar** in a patient with

229

thyrotoxicosis. Subtotal thyroidectomy is one of the options in treating thyrotoxicosis, the others being anti-thyroid drugs such as carbimazole, radioactive iodine, and beta-blockers for symptomatic relief. Following thyroidectomy 80% of patients are euthyroid, 15% are hypothyroid, and 5% remain thyrotoxic.

2. Left exotropia and **mature cataract.** Sensory exotropia is the result of monocular or binocular visual impairment by acquired lesions such as cataract, corneal scarring or severe ptosis.

3. Right iris abnormality, **left corneal scarring**, **mild left exotropia**, **hypertelorism** (increased interorbital distance), **broad nasal bridge** and **nose**, **maxillary hypoplasia**, and **abnormal dentition**. All these are features of Rieger syndrome.

4. Retinitis pigmentosa (RP), **macular hole**, and **disc cupping.** A true macular hole is incidental, although some patients with RP have chronic cystoid macular oedema which may give rise to a lamellar hole due to breakdown of cystoid spaces. About 3% of patients with RP have open-angle glaucoma.

5. Terrien marginal corneal degeneration and **perforation with iris prolapse**, which is a rare complication that may occur spontaneously or following trauma. More frequent problems are astigmatism, formation of pseudo-pterygia, and recurrent pain and inflammation.

6. Old inferior branch vein occlusion and **shunts**, and **recent cilioretinal arterial occlusion.** Collateral venous channels, characterized by slightly tortuous vessels, may develop locally or across the horizontal arcade between the superior and inferior vascular arcades. Other signs of old venous occlusion are hard exudate formation, and venous sheathing and sclerosis. It is rare for venous and arterial occlusion to be present in the same eye.

QUESTION 144

What have these conditions in common?

They are all cystic lesions

1. Primary iris cyst is a rare curiosity that usually arises from the iris epithelium. The vast majority are innocuous and asymptomatic. Rarely they become dislodged into the anterior chamber.

2. Microcystoid degeneration consists of tiny vesicles with indistinct boundaries on a greyish-white background which make the retina appear thickened and less transparent. The degeneration always starts adjacent to the ora serrata and extends circumferentially and posteriorly with a smooth undulating posterior border. The condition is present in all adult eyes, increasing in severity with age, and is not in itself causally related to RD – although it may give rise to retinoschisis.

3. Vitreous cyst is a rare congenital remnant of the primary hyaloidal system or ciliary body pigment epithelium. Most are asymptomatic and treatment is seldom required, although laser photocystotomy or vitrectomy have been suggested in patients with annoying symptoms.

4. Sinus mucocele develops when the drainage of normal para-nasal sinus secretions is obstructed due to infection, allergy, trauma, tumour or congenital narrowing. A slowly expanding cystic accumulation of mucoid secretions and epithelial debris develops and gradually erodes the bony walls of the sinuses, causing symptoms by encroaching upon surrounding tissues. Orbital invasion occurs usually from frontal or ethmoidal mucoceles. CT shows thinning of the bony walls of the sinus and a soft tissue mass which may displace the globe.

5. Cyst of Moll (apocrine hidrocystoma) is a round, non-tender, translucent, fluid-filled lesion on the anterior lid margin.

6. Secondary retinal cyst may develop in eyes with long-standing retinal detachment.

QUESTION 145

Which is the odd one out?

2 Shallow anterior chamber

All other signs occur in **pigment dispersion syndrome**: Krukenberg spindle (**1**); pigment granules on the iris surface and partial loss of the pupillary ruff (**3**); glaucomatous cupping may occur in pigmentary glaucoma (**4**); radial slit-like iris transillumination defects (**5**); very deep anterior chamber and posterior bowing of the peripheral iris demonstrated on high frequency ultrasonography (**6**). Pigment dispersion syndrome is characterized by the liberation of pigment granules from the iris pigment epithelium and their deposition throughout the anterior segment. Pigmentary obstruction of the trabecular spaces and damage to the trabeculum leads to elevation of intraocular pressure in a significant percentage of cases (pigmentary glaucoma).

QUESTION 146

Plant, fruit or mineral?

1. Plant – flower-shaped ('rosette') cataract may occur as a result of blunt trauma. It may subsequently disappear, remain stationary or progress to maturity.

2. Mineral – central Schnyder (crystalline) dystrophy is an AD condition which presents in the second decade with visual impairment and glare. It is characterized by a central, oval, subepithelial 'crystalline' opacity.

3. Plant – Christmas tree cataract is an uncommon age-related opacity characterized by striking, polychromatic, needle-like deposits in the deep cortex and nucleus.

4. Mineral – high-water marks are pigmented demarcation lines which develop at the junction of flat and detached retina in eyes with long-standing inferior retinal detachments.

5. Fruit – strawberry naevus (capillary haemangioma) presents soon after birth and most frequently affects the upper eyelid. It grows for 3–6 months after presentation and then involutes slowly. About 30% resolve by the age of 3 years and 70% by the age of 7 years.

6. Plant – morning glory anomaly is a very rare, usually unilateral sporadic condition that has a spectrum of severity. Typically it is characterized by a large disc with a funnel-shaped excavation surrounded by an annulus of chorioretinal disturbance. The blood vessels emerge from the rim of the excavation in a radial pattern like the spokes of a wheel.

QUESTION 147

What are these rare conditions?

1. Familial exudative vitreoretinopathy (Criswick–Schepens syndrome) is an AD slowly progressive condition characterized by fibrovascular proliferation in the temporal periphery and vitreoretinal traction resulting in ridge formation and 'dragging' of the disc. The appearance is very similar to retinopathy of prematurity but is not associated with low birth weight and patients are full-term.

2. Intrastromal corneal haemorrhage may rarely occur when non-perfused vessels in an eye with interstitial keratitis become re-perfused.

3. Fibrous dysplasia is a sporadic disorder characterized by expansible fibrous lesions within one or several bones that presents in childhood or early adult life. Orbital involvement may cause proptosis and displacement of the globe. It may be associated with McClune–Albright which also manifests café au lait spots and endocrine hyperfunction.

4. Multifocal vitelliform lesions may occasionally present in adult life and give rise to diagnostic problems. However, in these patients the EOG is normal and the family history is negative, unlike true juvenile Best macular dystrophy.

5. Complete cryptophthalmos is characterized by replacement of the eyelids by layer of skin which is fused with a microphthalmic eye. Incomplete cryptophthalmos is characterized by microphthalmos, rudimentary lids, and a small conjunctival sac.

6. Retinoblastoma invading the anterior segment is rare and tends to occur in older patients. It may cause a red eye due to tumour-induced uveitis, as well as iris nodules which may be associated with pseudo-hypopyon.

QUESTION 148

What are these surgical complications?

1. Surgically-induced scleritis following trabeculectomy. The scleritis typically starts within 3 weeks of the surgical procedure, but much longer intervals have been reported. It may be induced by any type of surgery including strabismus repair and scleral buckling for retinal detachment. The necrotizing process starts at the site of surgery and then extends outwards but, unlike other forms of necrotizing disease, it tends to remain localized to one segment.

2. Iris prolapse is very rare following small incision cataract surgery, but may occur when the incision is large.

3. Erosion of an Arruga suture which was used in the past for encirclement in retinal detachment surgery. Cheese-wiring of the sclera was a serious complication, which occurred when the suture was tied too tightly.

4. Laser pitting of IOL may occur when the laser beam is incorrectly focused. Although undesirable, a few laser marks on the IOL do not alter visual function or impair ocular tolerance of the implant.

5. Expulsive haemorrhage is a bleed into the suprachoroidal space which may result in extrusion of intraocular contents or apposition of retinal surfaces. It is a dreaded but rare complication of intraocular surgery. The source of the bleeding is a ruptured long or short posterior ciliary artery. Although the exact cause is unknown, contributing factors include advanced age, glaucoma, increased axial length, systemic cardiovascular disease, and vitreous loss. Ultrasonography is useful in assessing severity.

6. Extrusion of an orbital implant following enucleation may occur if the implant is too large and if Tenon fascia has not been meticulously sutured. The risk of extrusion is further increased with prior irradiation and infection.

QUESTION 149

What have these conditions in common?

They are all pre-malignant conditions

1. Cutaneous horn may overly an area of epidermis that is dysplastic or shows evidence of squamous cell carcinoma. It is a clinical marker that the underlying epidermis is abnormal rather than a diagnosis in itself. It is therefore necessary to biopsy the lesion, and if invasive squamous cell carcinoma has developed, wide excision should be performed.

2. Lentigo maligna (melanoma *in-situ*, intraepidermal melanoma, Hutchinson freckle and precancerous melanosis of Dubreuilh) is a relatively uncommon condition that develops in sun-damaged skin of elderly individuals that may subsequently infiltrate the dermis and become malignant. It is characterized by a very slowly expanding pigmented macule with an irregular border. Nodular thickening and areas of irregular pigmentation are highly suggestive of malignant transformation.

3. Actinic (solar, senile) keratosis is a slowly-growing lesion that typically affects elderly individuals who have been exposed to excessive sunlight. It has a potential for transformation into squamous cell carcinoma and is characterized by a hyperkeratotic plaque.

4. Conjunctival intraepithelial neoplasia is an uncommon, slowly progressive unilateral disease which has no pathognomonic characteristic, although a limbal location is most common. The lesion may be gelatinous, papillary, nodular or leukoplakic with an overlying white keratin plaque. Histology is required to determine if the lesion is dysplastic, a carcinoma *in situ*, or a squamous cell carcinoma.

5. Xeroderma pigmentosum is an AR disease characterized by skin damage on exposure to natural sunlight which gives rise to progressive cutaneous pigmentation abnormalities. Affected patients have a bird-like facies and a great propensity to the development of skin basal cell carcinoma, squamous cell carcinoma, and melanoma, which may be multiple. Conjunctival malignancies have also been reported.

6. Primary acquired melanosis (PAM) is an uncommon, almost always unilateral condition which typically affects middle-aged whites. It is characterized by irregular areas of flat, brown intraepithelial pigmentation, which may involve any part of the conjunctiva. There are two histological types: PAM without melanocytic cellular atypia, which is benign, and PAM with atypia, which has a 50% chance of transformation into infiltrating melanoma within 5 years.

QUESTION 150

Match the clinical sign (1–3) with the angiogram (A–C)

1 and C

Thyrotoxicosis is frequently associated with goitre (**1**). Thyroid ophthalmopathy may give rise to soft tissue involvement, lid retraction, proptosis, restrictive myopathy, and optic neuropathy. Choroidal folds are a series of roughly parallel alternating light and dark delicate lines or striae which are most frequently noted at the posterior pole and which may occur in a wide variety of orbital lesions including thyroid ophthalmopathy. On **FA** the crests of the folds are hyperfluorescent as a result of increased background choroidal fluorescence showing through the stretched and thinned RPE, and the troughs are hypofluorescent due to blockage by compressed and thickened RPE (**C**).

2 and A

High myopia is defined as an axial length of the globe over 26 mm. In some cases the length may be very much longer and apparent clinically as prominent enlargement of the globe (**2**). **FA** in degenerative myopia shows areas of choroidal hypofluorescence due to loss of the choriocapillaris, and enhanced visualization of residual larger choroidal vessels (**A**).

3 and B

Relapsing polychondritis is a rare idiopathic condition characterized by small vessel vasculitis involving cartilage resulting in recurrent, often progressive, inflammatory episodes involving multiple organ systems. Collapse of the nasal cartilage resulting in a 'saddle-shaped' deformity is characteristic (**3**). It is an important cause of scleritis which may be non-necrotizing or necrotizing. **FA** of the latter shows extensive areas of non-perfusion (**B**).

Section 4

Questions 151 to 200. Answers start on page 286.

Q **151** What is the inheritance pattern of this condition?

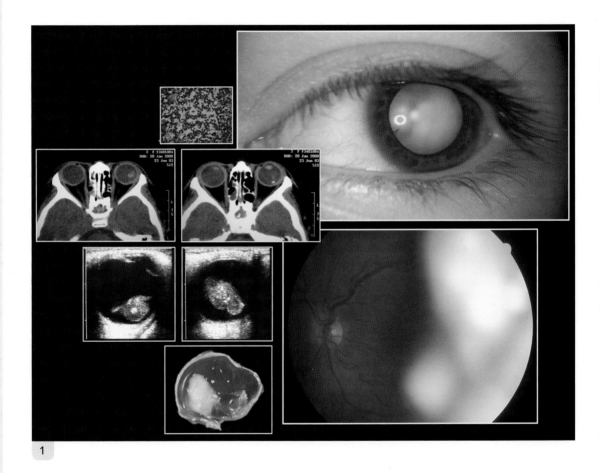

1

Answer on page 286

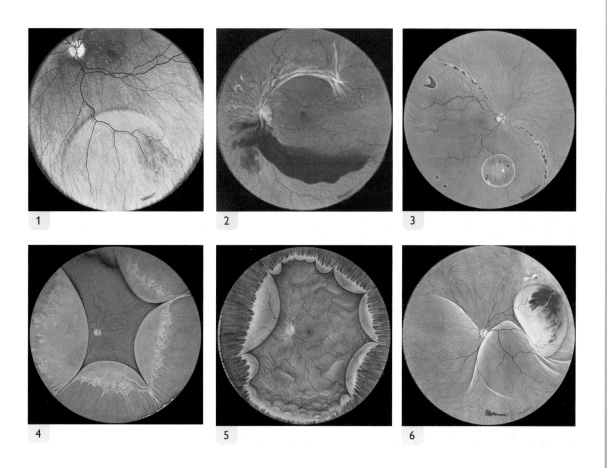

1

2

3

4

5

6

Answer on pages 286–287

Q 153 What are these rare conditions?

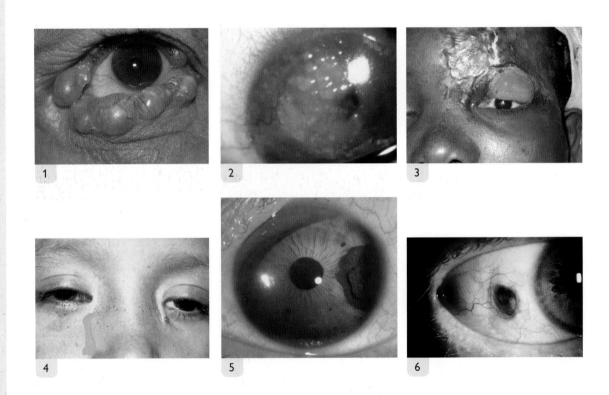

Answer on page 287

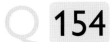

Match the radiographs (1–3) with the eye (A–C)

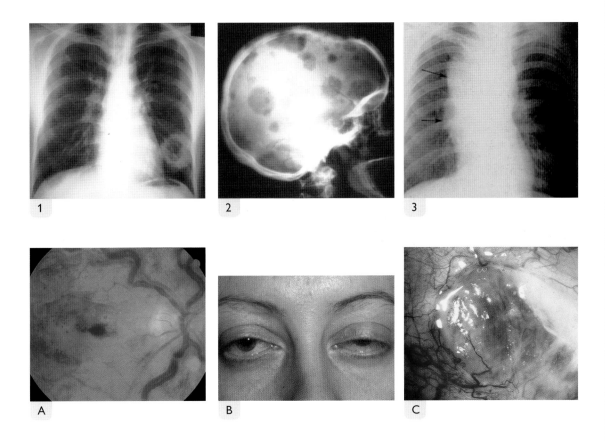

Answer on pages 287–288

Q 155 What multiple conditions are present?

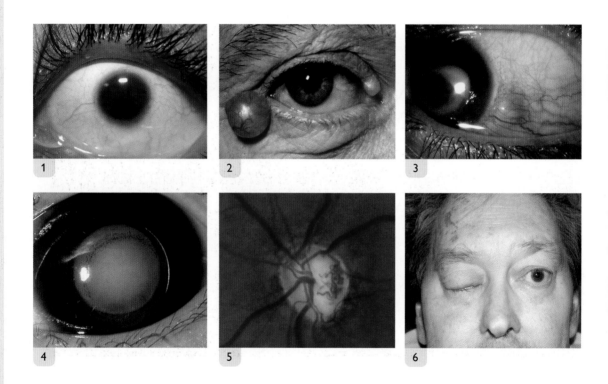

Answer on page 288

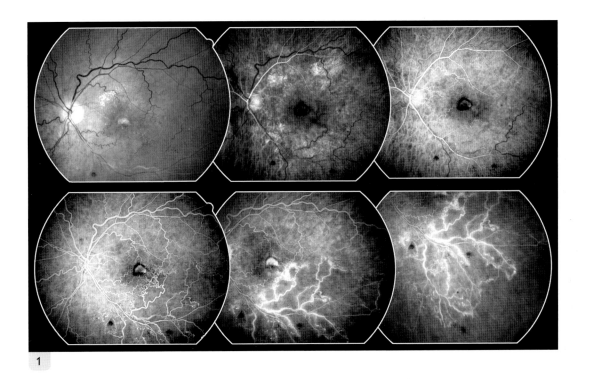

Q **156** What double pathology is present?

Answer on page 288

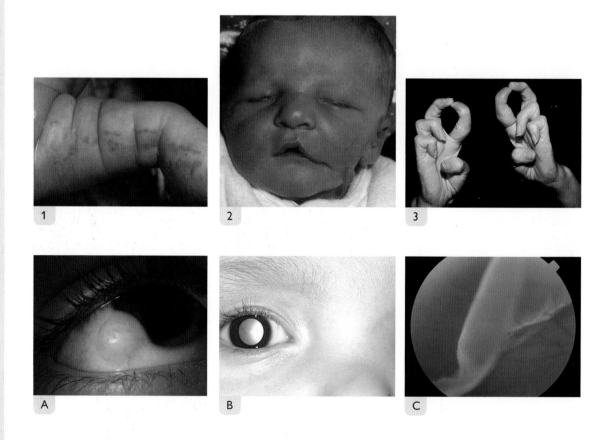

Q 157 Match the systemic feature (1–3) with the eye (A–C)

Answer on pages 288–289

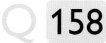

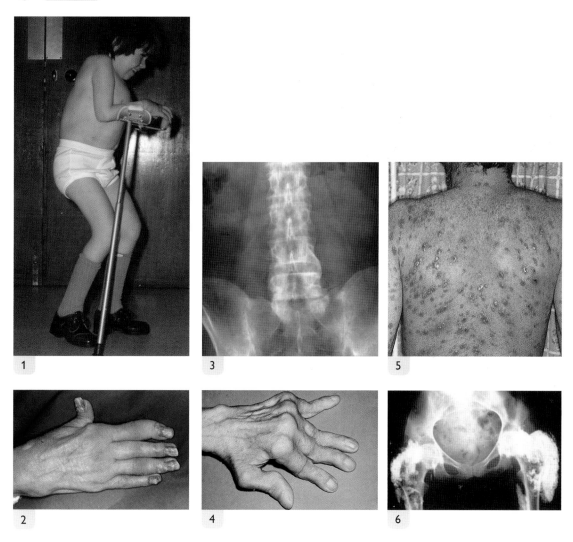

Q **158** Which conditions are not associated with anterior uveitis?

1

2

3

4

5

6

Answer on pages 289–290

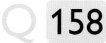

Q 159 What are these subtle signs in posterior uveitis?

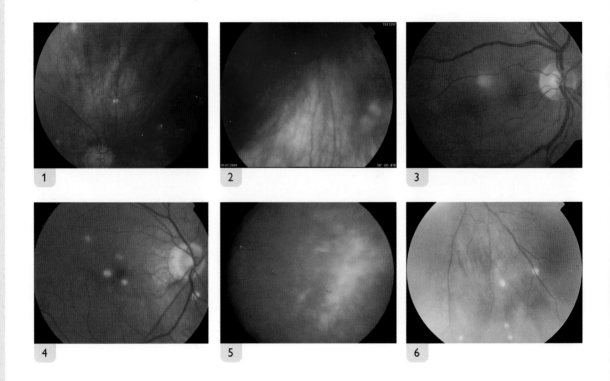

Answer on page 290

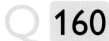
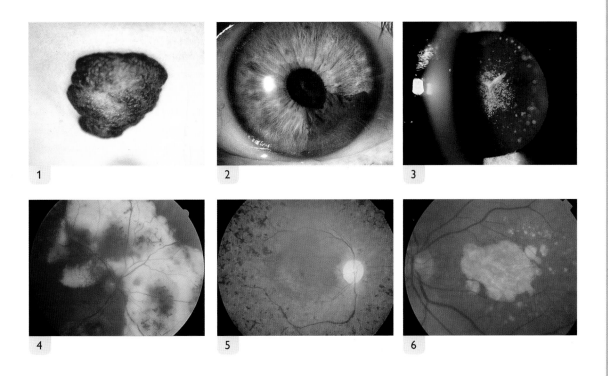

Answer on pages 290–291

245

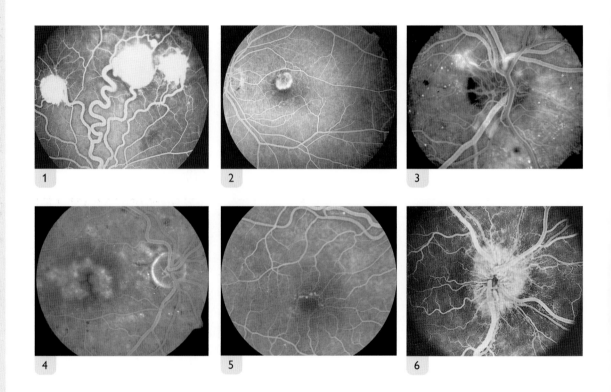

Q 161 What are the complications of these conditions?

Answer on pages 291–292

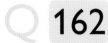What have these conditions in common?

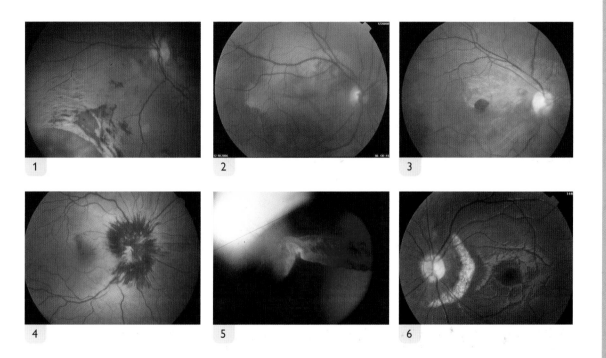

1

2

3

4

5

6

Answer on page 292

Answer on page 292

Q **163** What are these eponymous conditions?

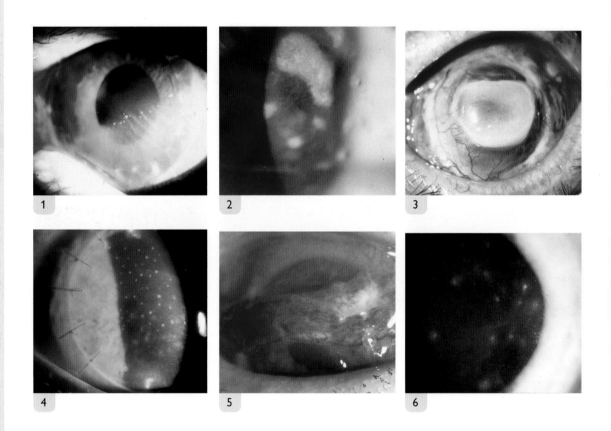

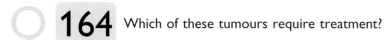

Q **164** Which of these tumours require treatment?

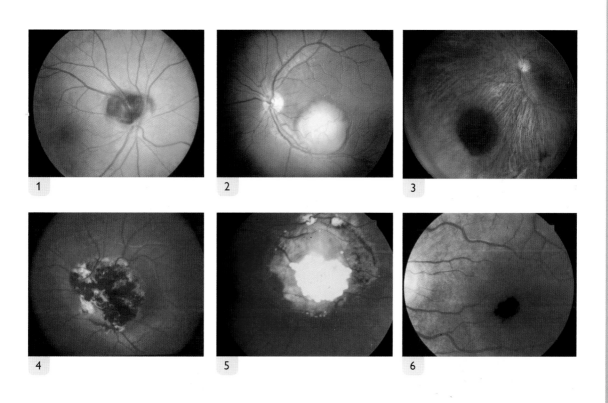

1

2

3

4

5

6

Answer on page 293

Q 165 What are the ocular manifestations of these syndromic conditions?

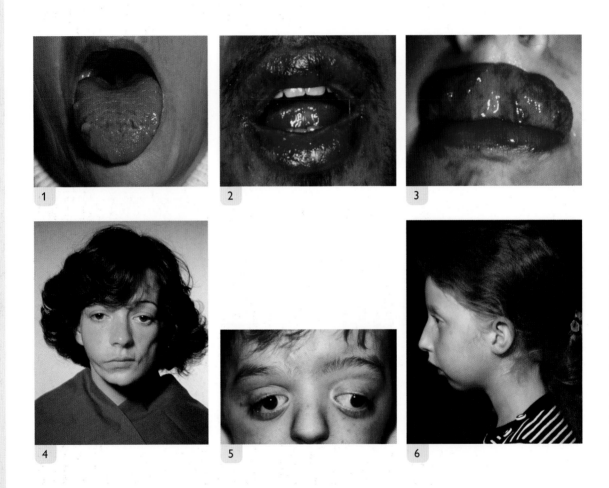

Answer on pages 293–294

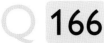

Q 166 What are the main ocular manifestations of these systemic conditions?

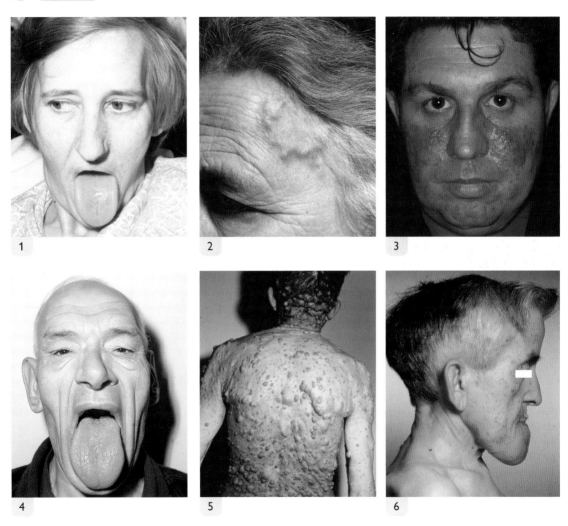

1

2

3

4

5

6

Answer on page 294

Q **167** What vision-threatening complications may these conditions cause?

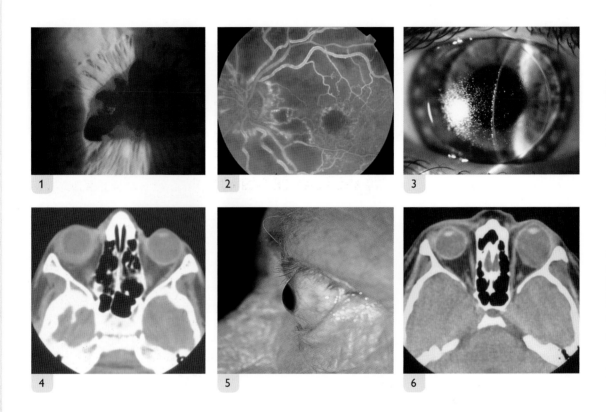

1

2

3

4

5

6

Answer on page 295

Q **168** What treatment has been performed?

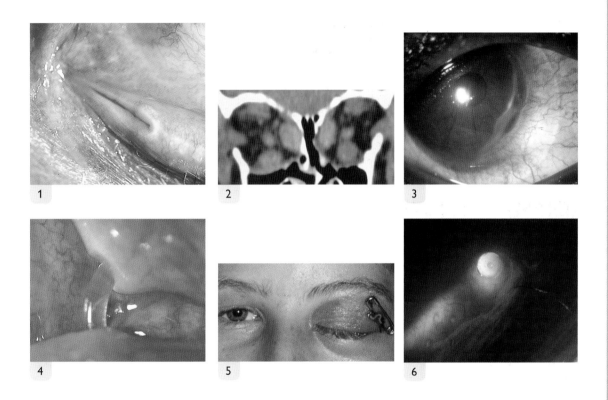

1

2

3

4

5

6

Answer on pages 295–296

What treatment has been performed and was it successful? (A = before, B = after treatment)

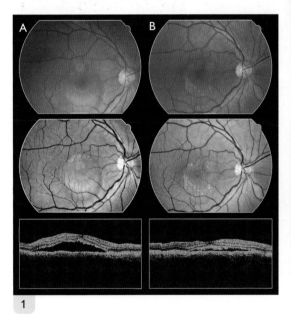

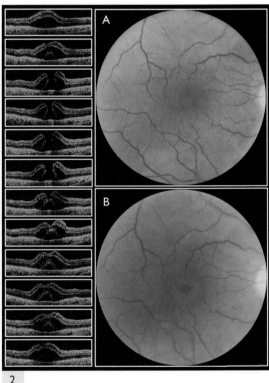

Answer on page 296

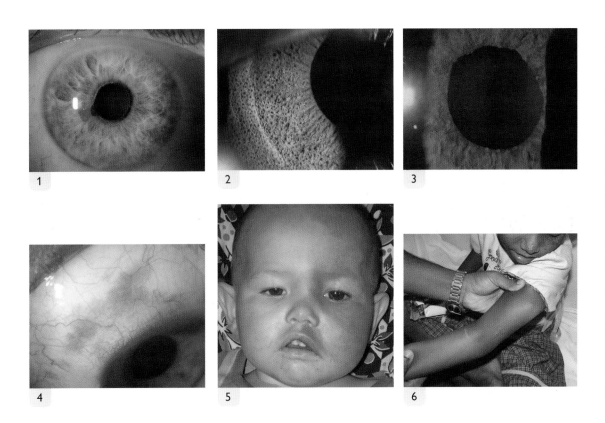

1

2

3

4

5

6

Answer on page 296

Q 171 Which investigation would be appropriate for these conditions?

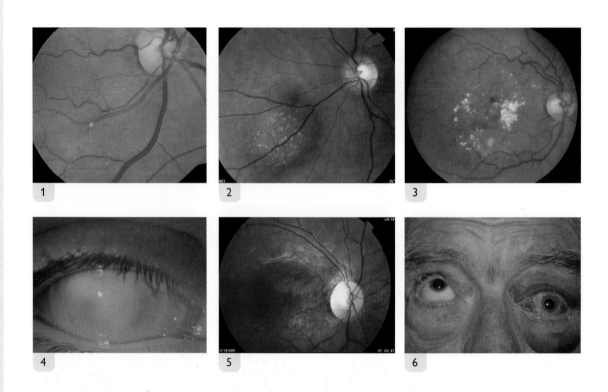

Answer on page 297

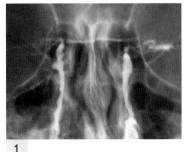
172 What are these investigations?

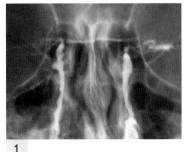

1

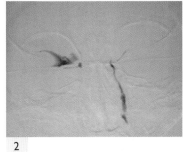

2

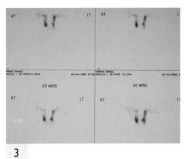

3

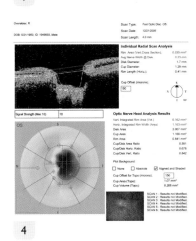

4

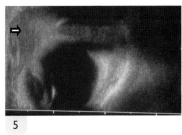

5

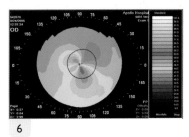

6

Answer on pages 297–298

Q 173 What treatment has been performed?

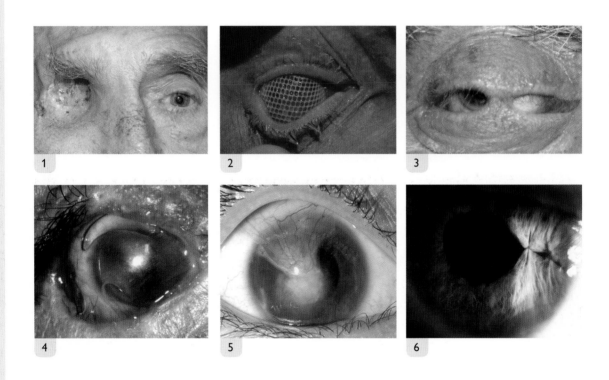

Answer on page 298

Q 174 Match the motility defect (1–3) with the scan (A–C)

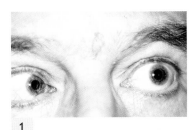

1

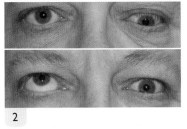

2

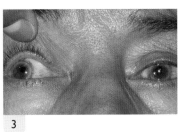

3

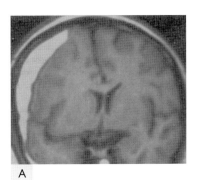

A

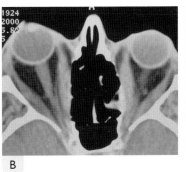

B

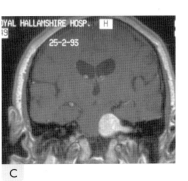

C

Answer on pages 298–299

Q **175** What is the diagnosis?

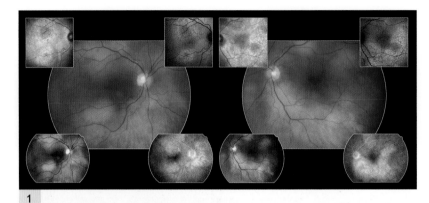

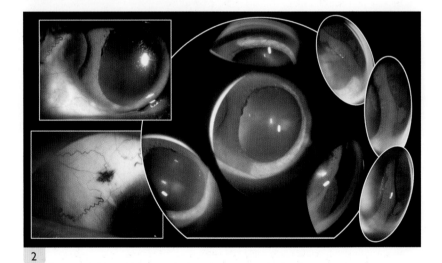

Answer on page 299

Q 176 What is the diagnosis?

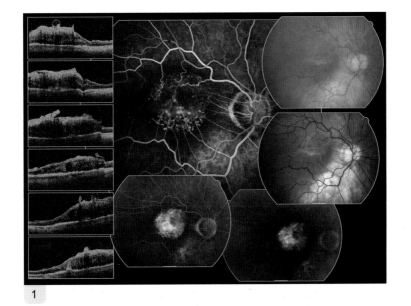

1

2

Answer on page 299

Q 177 What is this condition?

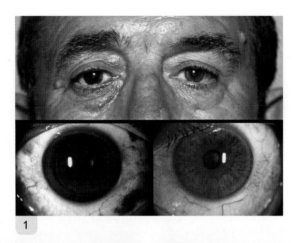

1

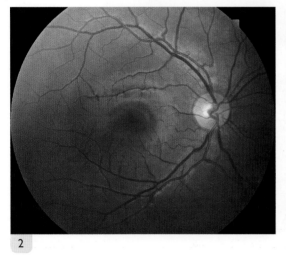

2

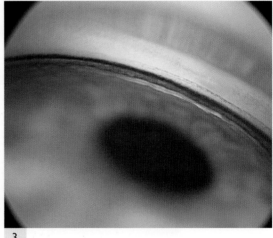

3

Answer on pages 299–300

Q 178 Match the fundus (1–3) with the ERG (A–C)

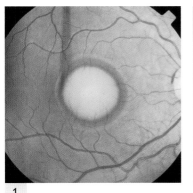

1

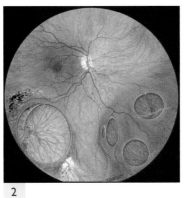

2

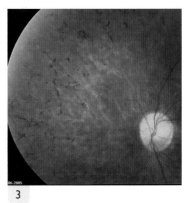

3

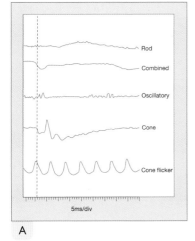

A

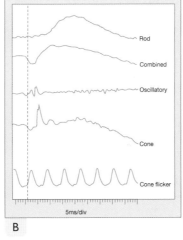

B

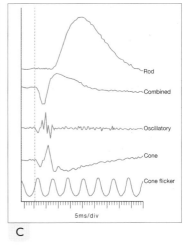

C

Answer on page 300

Q 179 What are these rare congenital conditions?

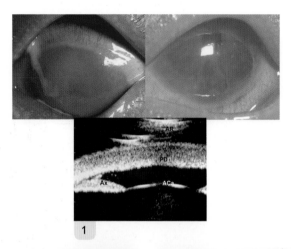

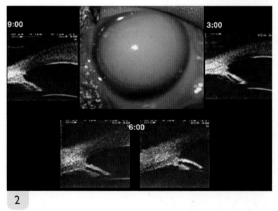

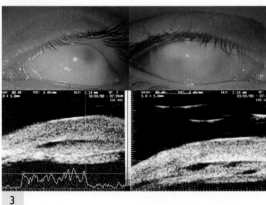

Answer on page 300

Q **180** What are these eponymous conditions?

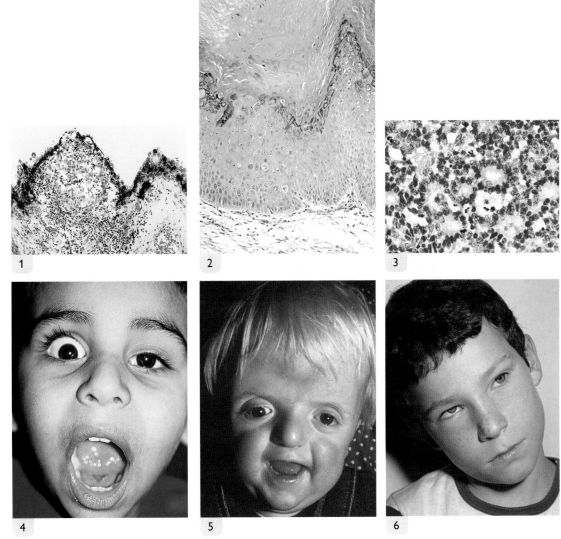

Answer on pages 300–301

Q 181 What are these inherited conditions?

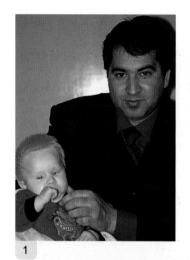

1

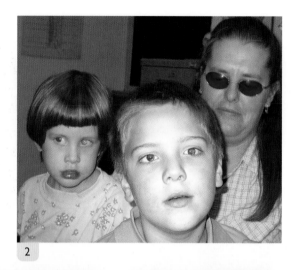

2

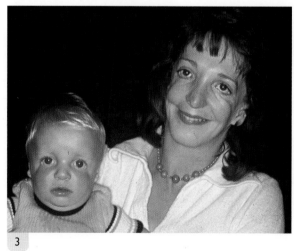

3

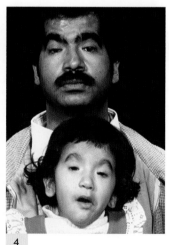

4

Answer on page 301

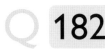

What are the presenting symptoms of these conditions?

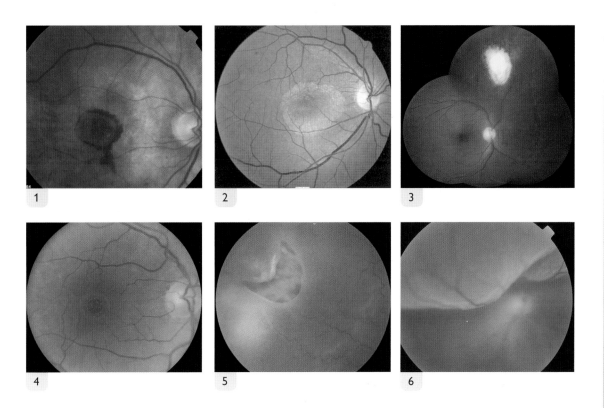

Answer on pages 301–302

Q 183 What multiple signs are present?

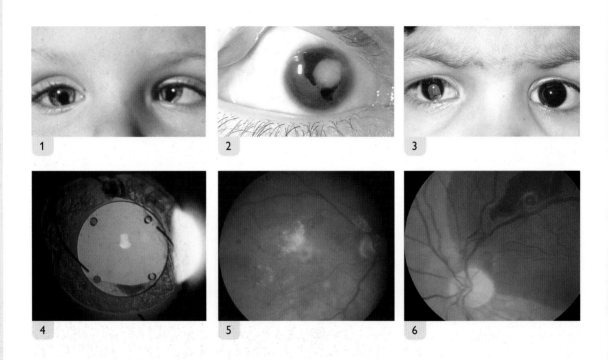

Answer on page 302

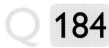
Q **184** Match the diabetic maculopathy (1–3) with the angiogram (A–C)

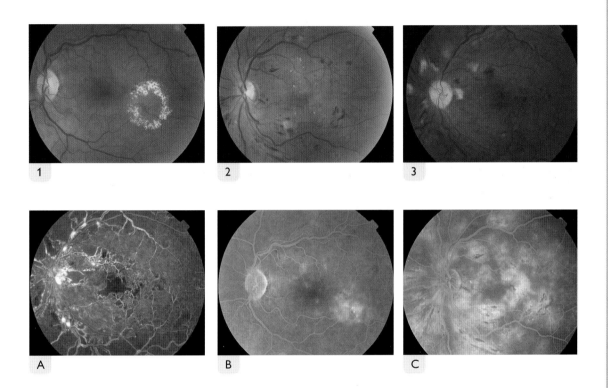

Answer on page 302

Q **185** What are these rare acquired conditions?

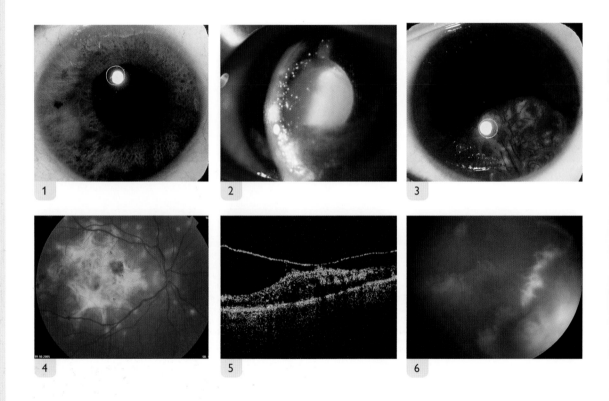

1
2
3
4
5
6

Answer on page 303

Q 186 What are these rare congenital conditions?

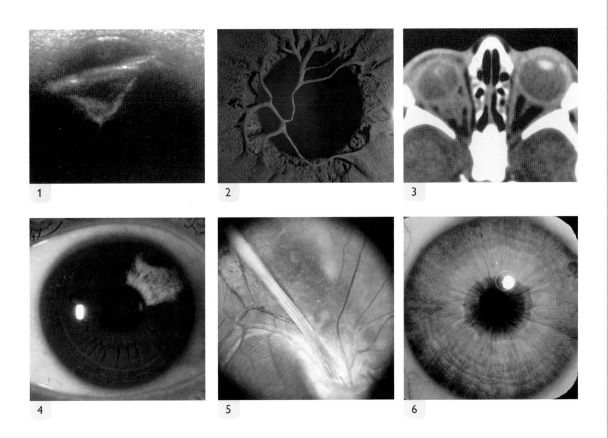

1

2

3

4

5

6

Answer on pages 303–304

Q **187** Match the clinical signs (1–3) with the histology (A–C)

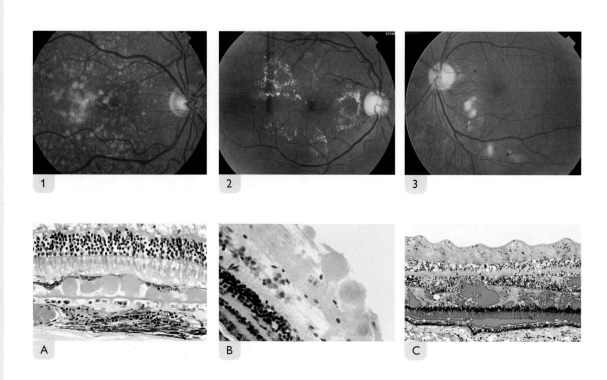

Answer on page 304

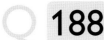
Which of these intraocular tumours may be bilateral?

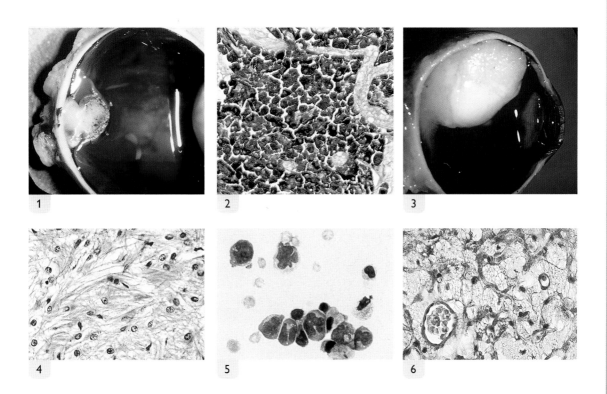

Answer on page 304

273

Q 189 What treatment has been performed?

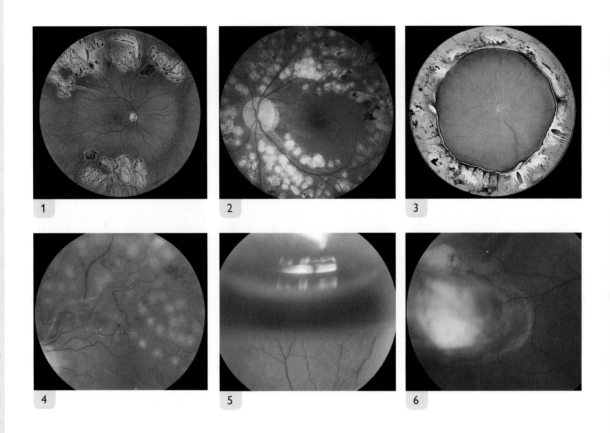

Answer on pages 304–305

Q **190** What are these conditions involving the anterior chamber?

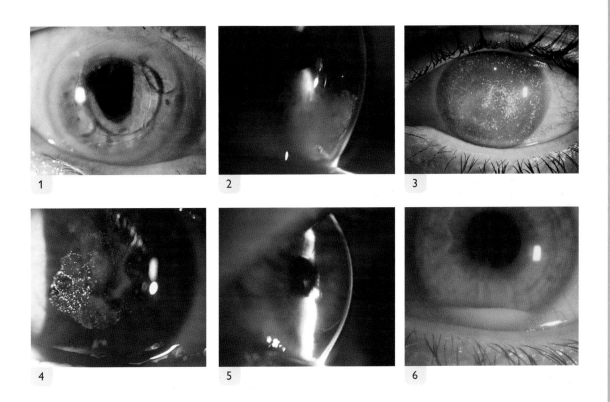

1

2

3

4

5

6

Answer on pages 305–306

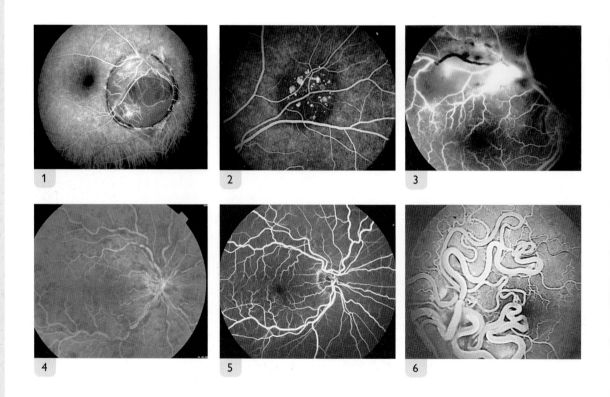

Q 191 What do these angiograms show?

Answer on page 306

Q **192** What is this disease?

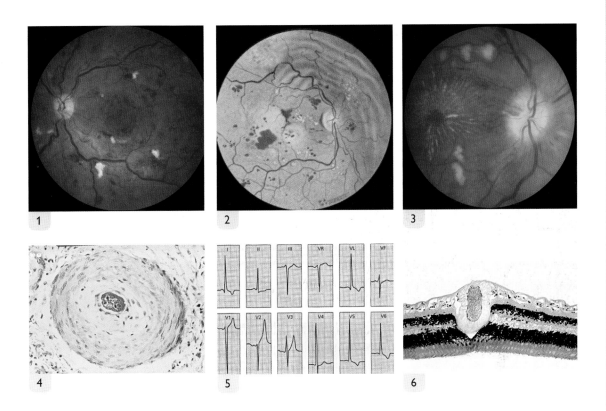

Answer on page 306

Are these conditions unilateral or bilateral?

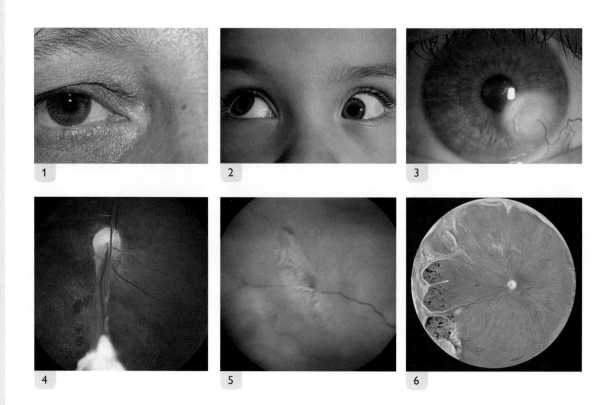

Answer on pages 306–307

Q **194** Match the eye (1–3) with the teeth (A–C)

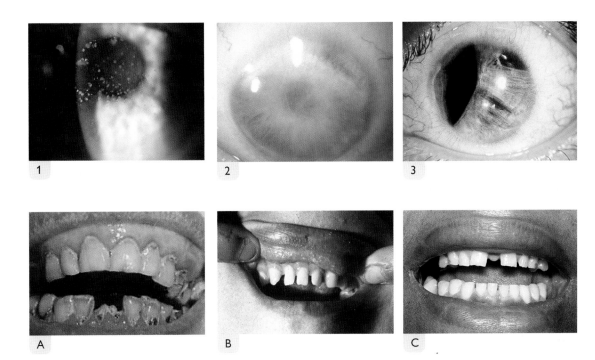

Answer on page 307

Q 195 Systemic treatment with immunosuppressives or antivirals?

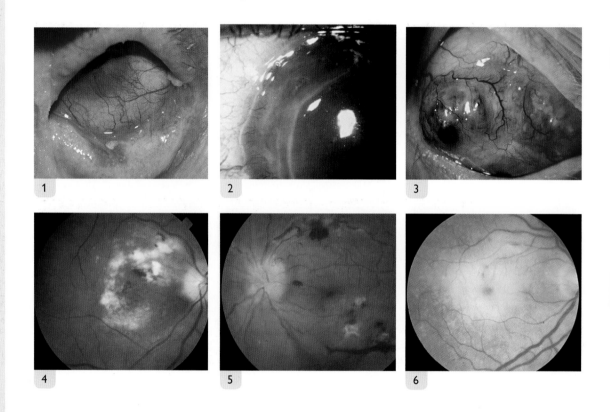

Answer on pages 307–308

Q 196   Topical treatment with steroids, antivirals or antibiotics?

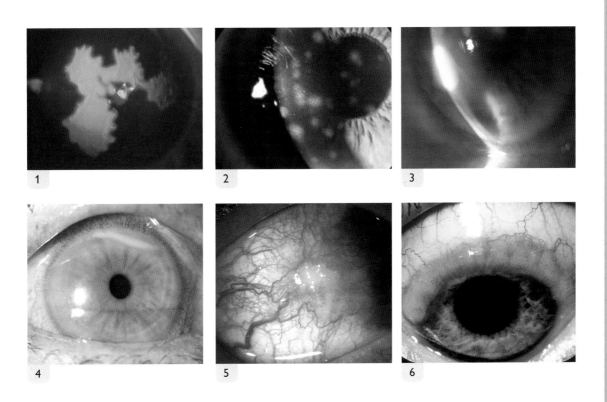

Answer on page 308

Q 197 What are these congenital conditions?

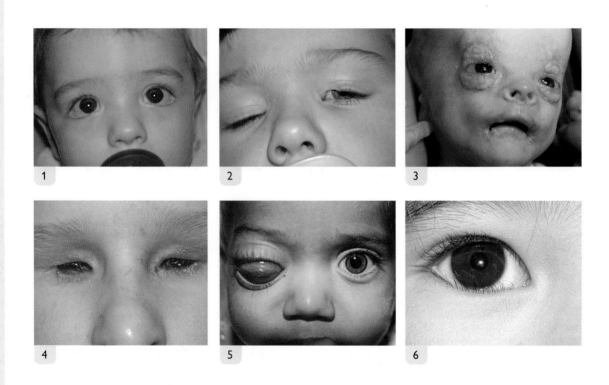

1

2

3

4

5

6

Answer on pages 308–309

198 What is the mode of inheritance?

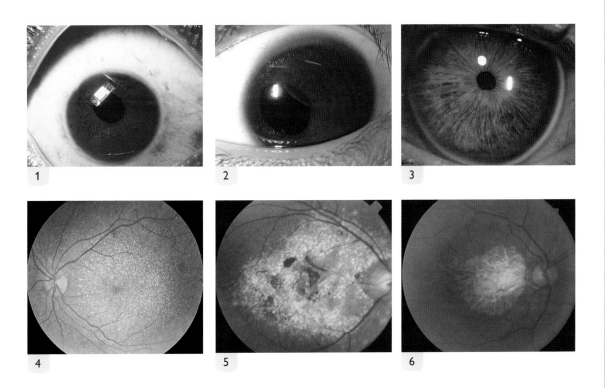

Answer on page 309

199 Match the corneal ectasia (1–3) with the map (A–C)

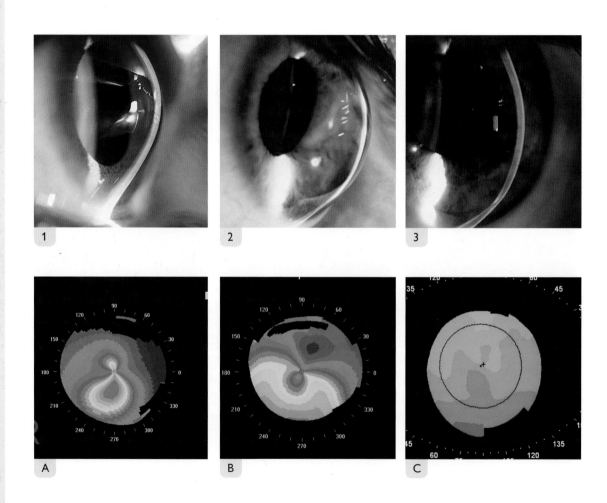

Answer on pages 309–310

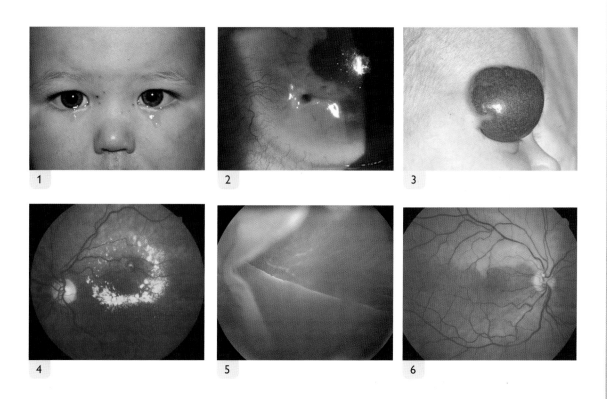

Answer on page 310

QUESTION 151

What is the inheritance pattern of this condition?

Retinoblastoma may be heritable or non-heritable. The predisposing gene to retinoblastoma (RB1) is at 13q14. Heritable (germline) retinoblastoma accounts for 40% in which one allele of the *RB1* (a tumour suppressor gene) is mutated in all body cells. When a further mutagenic event ('second hit') affects the second allele, the cell undergoes malignant transformation. Because all the retinal precursor cells contain the initial mutation, these children develop bilateral and multifocal tumours. The mutation is transmitted in 50% but because of incomplete penetrance only 40% of offspring will be affected. If a child has heritable retinoblastoma, the risk to siblings is 2% if the parents are healthy, and 40% if a parent is affected. About 15% of patients with hereditary retinoblastoma manifest unilateral involvement. Non-heritable (somatic) retinoblastoma accounts for the remaining 60% of cases. The tumour is unilateral and not transmissible. If a patient has a solitary retinoblastoma and no positive family history, this is probably but not definitely non-heritable so that the risk in each sibling and offspring is about 1%.

QUESTION 152

Retinal detachment or simulating lesion?

1. Acquired retinoschisis is characterized by a convex, smooth, thin, and relatively immobile elevation. Retinal breaks may be absent or present in one or both leaves. The thin inner leaf of the schisis cavity may be mistaken, on cursory examination, for an atrophic long-standing rhegmatogenous RD but demarcation lines and secondary cysts in the inner leaf are absent.

2. Tractional retinal detachment lacks retinal breaks and has a relatively immobile concave configuration. The subretinal fluid is less deep than in a rhegmatogenous RD and seldom extends to the ora serrata. The highest elevation of the retina occurs at sites of vitreoretinal traction. If a tractional RD develops a break it assumes the characteristics of a rhegmatogenous RD and progresses more quickly (combined tractional-rhegmatogenous RD).

3. Rhegmatogenous retinal detachment has one or more retinal breaks, a convex configuration, and a slightly opaque and corrugated appearance. The subretinal fluid extends up to the ora serrata. Features of long-standing cases are retinal thinning, secondary intraretinal cysts, and subretinal demarcation lines (high-water marks).

4. Choroidal detachment is usually associated with a low intraocular pressure. The elevations are brown, convex, smooth and relatively immobile, and also involve the ciliary body. Temporal and nasal bullae tend to be most prominent. The elevations do not extend to the posterior pole because they are limited by the firm adhesion between the suprachoroidal lamellae where the vortex veins enter their scleral canals.

5. Uveal effusion syndrome is a rare, idiopathic condition which most frequently affects middle-aged hypermetropic men. It is characterized by ciliochoroidal detachment followed by exudative RD which may be bilateral. Uveal effusion may be mistaken for a RD complicated by choroidal detachment or a ring melanoma of the anterior choroid.

6. Exudative retinal detachment lacks retinal breaks and has a smooth convex configuration. The detached retina is very mobile and exhibits the phenomenon of 'shifting fluid' in which SRF responds to the force of gravity and detaches the area of retina under which it accumulates. The cause of the RD, such as a choroidal tumour, may be apparent, or the patient may have an associated systemic disease responsible for the RD (e.g. Harada disease, toxaemia of pregnancy).

QUESTION 153

What are these rare conditions?

1. Multiple apocrine hidrocystomas (cysts of Moll) are filled with clear or milky fluid and have a shiny smooth overlying skin. Multiple lesions are thought to represent an ectodermal dysplasia which also manifests hypodontia, palmar-plantar hyperkeratosis, and onychodystrophy.

2. Gelatinous corneal dystrophy is a rare AR condition characterized by mulberry-like lesions consisting of amyloid. It is seen mainly in Japan.

3. Cicatricial ectropion of the upper eyelid due to severe scarring caused by herpes zoster ophthalmicus.

4. Lacrimal sac fistula demonstrated with fluorescein. Congenital fistulae may be left untreated unless they allow flow of tears onto the face. Acquired fistulae may occasionally follow inappropriate treatment of dacryocystitis.

5. Iris melanocytoma is a deeply-pigmented nodular mass with a mossy, granular surface and absence of intrinsic vasculature, often involving the iris root. It may undergo spontaneous necrosis resulting in seeding of the iris stroma and chamber angle.

6. Scleral hyaline plaque typically occurs asymptomatically in the interpalpebral region, close to the insertion of the horizontal rectus muscles. Rarely, they may cut through the conjunctiva and require removal.

QUESTION 154

Match the radiographs (1–3) with the eye (A–C)

I and C

Wegener granulomatosis is an idiopathic, multisystem granulomatous disorder characterized by generalized small vessel vasculitis affecting predominantly the respiratory tract and kidneys. It affects males more commonly than females. Lower respiratory tract involvement may result in nodular lesions, infiltrates, and cavities with fluid levels (**1**). The disease may be associated with rapidly progressive, necrotizing granulomatous scleritis (**C**).

2 and A

Multiple myeloma is a rare malignant disease caused by proliferation of plasma cells in the bone marrow with the production of characteristic monoclonal M protein in blood and urine. It is characterized by osteolytic bony lesions (**2**) that cause pain, fractures, and hypercalcaemia. Retinopathy characterized by retinal haemorrhages, and venous dilatation, tortuosity, and segmentation (**A**) is uncommon.

3 and B

Myasthenia gravis is an autoimmune disease in which there is antibody mediate damage and destruction of acetylcholine receptors in striated muscle. The resultant impairment of neuromuscular conduction causes weakness and fatigue of skeletal musculature. Myasthenia may be ocular, bulbar or generalized. Thymoma (**3**) is present in 10% of cases. Patients under the age of 40 years without thymoma generally have a hyperplastic thymus but in older patients the thymus is usually normal (atrophic). Presentation is most commonly in the third decade, most frequently with ptosis (**B**) or diplopia which may be worse towards the end of the day.

QUESTION 155

What multiple conditions are present?

1. Microphthalmos and **iris coloboma.** Microphthalmos is a unilateral or bilateral developmental arrest of ocular growth, defined as total axial length at least 2 standard deviations below age-similar controls. Simple microphthalmos is not associated with other major ocular malformations. Complex (colobomatous) microphthalmos is associated with coloboma, usually of the iris.

2. Cyst of Moll (apocrine hidrocystoma) and **eccrine hidrocystoma.** The former is located on the lid margin, and the latter is located laterally and does not involve the lid margin itself.

3. Acanthamoeba keratitis and **scleritis.** The ring abscess is typical of acanthamoeba; scleral involvement may develop as extension of keratitis, or independently.

4. Microspherophakia and **congenital cataract.** Microspherophakia may occur in isolation or in association with Weill–Marchesani syndrome and Marfan syndrome. Co-existing cataract is rare.

5. Glaucomatous cupping and **disc shunts.** The latter are uncommon and may join the central vein with parapapillary veins, or two retinal veins.

6. Ptosis and **scarring from herpes zoster ophthalmicus.** It is likely that the ptosis is due to associated third nerve palsy.

QUESTION 156

What double pathology is present?

The FA shows a small spot of progressive hyperfluorescence at the macula from a **choroidal neovascular membrane** surrounded by hypofluorescence due to blockage by blood, as well as capillary nonperfusion and staining of veins due to an old inferotemporal **retinal branch vein occlusion**.

QUESTION 157

Match the systemic feature (1–3) with the eye (A–C)

I and B

Bloch–Sulzberger syndrome (incontinentia pigmenti) is a rare XLD disorder that is lethal *in utero* for boys. It is characterized by a vesciculobullous rash on the trunk and extremities (**1**). About one-third of patients have retinal dysplasia which may give rise to leukocoria (**B**).

2 and A

Goldenhar syndrome is a sporadic condition characterized by preauricular appendages, mandibular hypoplasia, variable clefting (**2**), and hemivertebrae. Epibulbar dermoids (**A**), which may be bilateral, are common. Upper lid colobomas may also occur.

3 and C

Ehlers–Danlos syndrome type 6 (ocular sclerotic) is a rare, usually AR disorder of collagen caused by deficiency of procollagen lysyl hydroxylase. There are 9 distinct subtypes but only type 6, and rarely type 4, are associated with ocular features. The skin is thin and hyperelastic, and joints hypermobile (**3**). High myopia and retinal detachment (**C**) are common ocular associations.

QUESTION 158

Which conditions are not associated with anterior uveitis?

1. Juvenile idiopathic arthritis is an inflammatory arthritis of at least 6 weeks duration occurring before the age of 16 years. It is by far the most common disease associated with childhood **chronic anterior uveitis**. Risk factors for uveitis include early-onset pauciarticular disease, and positive findings for antinuclear antibodies and HLA-DR 5.

2. Psoriatic arthritis affects both sexes equally and is associated with an increased prevalence of HLA-B27 and HLA-B17. Nail dystrophy is invariable, and some patients develop severe arthritis.

Anterior uveitis is uncommon. Other ocular manifestations include conjunctivitis, marginal keratitis, and secondary Sjögren syndrome.

3. Ankylosing spondylitis is characterized by inflammation, calcification, and ossification of ligaments and capsules of joints with resultant bony ankylosis of the axial skeleton. It typically affects males, 90% of whom are HLA-B27 positive. About 30% of patients develop recurrent attacks of **acute anterior uveitis**.

4. Rheumatoid arthritis is an autoimmune systemic disease characterized by a symmetrical, destructive, deforming, inflammatory polyarthropathy, in association with a spectrum of extra-articular manifestations and circulating antiglobulin antibodies. Involvement of the small joints of the hands is characteristic, and may give rise to serious deformity. Ocular manifestations are keratoconjunctivitis sicca, scleritis, and peripheral ulcerative keratitis, but **not uveitis**.

5. Syphilis is caused by the spirochaete *Treponema pallidum*. Primary syphilis occurs after an incubation period commonly lasting 2–4 weeks and is characterized by a painless ulcer (chancre) at the site of infection. Secondary syphilis usually develops 6–8 weeks after the chancre and is characterized by symmetrical maculopapular rash on the trunk, palms, and soles. **Anterior uveitis** occurs in about 4% of patients with secondary syphilis. It is usually acute and bilateral in 50% of cases.

6. Systemic sclerosis is an idiopathic, chronic connective tissue disease affecting the skin (scleroderma) and internal organs, occurring most commonly in females under the age of 50. Subcutaneous deposition of calcium (calcinosis cutis) is uncommon and may be detected on x-ray. Uveitis does **not occur**, although some patients develop tight eyelids, and rarely keratoconjunctivitis sicca, conjunctival forniceal shortening, nodular episcleritis, and cotton-wool spots in the fundus.

QUESTION 159

What are these subtle signs in posterior uveitis?

1. 'Histo' spots in presumed ocular histoplasmosis syndrome (POHS) consist of roundish, slightly irregular, yellowish-white lesions about 200 μm in diameter often associated with pigment clumps within or at the margins of the scars. The lesions are scattered in the mid-retinal periphery and posterior fundus. The main cause of visual morbidity is maculopathy due to choroidal neovascularization.

2. Snowballs in the vitreous together with snowbanking of the inferior pars plana is characteristic of active pars planitis, which is a subset of idiopathic intermediate uveitis (IU). The latter is an insidious, chronic, relapsing disease in which the vitreous is the major site of the inflammation. It may be idiopathic or associated with a systemic disease. Pars planitis occurs more commonly in children while other forms of IU occur in an older age group, reflecting an increase in systemic associations such as multiple sclerosis, sarcoidosis, and Lyme disease. The main cause of visual morbidity is chronic cystoid macular oedema.

3. Focal retinitis in early ocular candidiasis manifests as a small white lesion at the posterior pole. Subsequent extension into the vitreous results in vitritis which may be associated with 'cotton-ball' opacities, similar to snowballs in pars planitis. Untreated candida endophthalmitis results in visual loss due to retinal necrosis and retinal detachment.

4. Multiple, small, yellow-white spots at the level of the inner choroid involving the posterior pole all of the same age are characteristic of punctate inner choroidopathy which is an uncommon idiopathic disease that typically affects young myopic women. The main cause of visual morbidity is maculopathy due to choroidal neovascularization, which occurs in about 40% of cases.

5. Peripheral retinal opacification with overlying vitritis in early acute retinal necrosis which is a rare but devastating viral retinitis that typically affects otherwise healthy individuals. The main causes of visual morbidity are retinal detachment and ischaemic optic neuropathy.

6. Multiple small, yellow-white peripheral lesions represent asymptomatic retinal granulomas in sarcoidosis.

QUESTION 160

At what age do these conditions present?

1. Capillary haemangioma (strawberry naevus) typically presents **soon after birth**.

2. Iris melanoma presents in the **fifth to sixth decades** of life, which is earlier than ciliary body and choroidal melanoma. The tumour is invariably located in the inferior half of the iris and often associated with surface vessels. Large tumours may cause distortion of the pupil, ectropion uveae, and localized lens opacities.

3. Sutural and fine dot lens opacities are present at **birth** but not usually diagnosed until later.

4. Coats disease presents between the ages of **5 and 10 years**. It is characterized by retinal telangiectasis and massive subretinal exudation. It is unilateral and principally affects boys.

5. Retinitis pigmentosa presents with nyctalopia, often in the **third decade**, but may be sooner depending on the pedigree. The initial findings are arteriolar narrowing and mild perivascular pigmentary changes. This is followed by coarse, 'bonespicule' pigmentation which gradually spreads and increases in intensity.

6. Dry age-related macular degeneration typically develops after the **seventh decade** of life. Presentation is with gradual deterioration of central vision. Both eyes are usually affected but not to the same extent. End-stage disease is characterized by geographic atrophy of the sensory retina, RPE, and choriocapillaris, often surrounded by drusen.

QUESTION 161

What are the complications of these conditions?

1. Retinal haemangioblastoma (capillary haemangioma) is characterized by early hyperfluorescence of the tumour due to filling followed by late leakage. Complications include exudate formation around the lesion as well as at the macula, bleeding and leakage resulting in macular oedema and exudative retinal detachment, fibrous band formation and tractional retinal detachment, vitreous haemorrhage, secondary glaucoma, and phthisis bulbi. Treatment options include laser photocoagulation, cryotherapy, brachytherapy, photodynamic therapy, and vitreoretinal surgery for advanced disease.

2. Choroidal neovascularization (CNV) is characterized by 'lacy' hyperfluorescence during the early phase of dye transit, bright fluorescence during peak transit, and then leakage and late staining. Important causes include wet age-related macular degeneration, certain inflammatory conditions of the choroid (e.g. punctate inner choroidopathy), high myopia, angioid streaks, and choroidal rupture. Complications of CNV include bleeding into the sub-RPE and subretinal space, hard exudate formation, macular oedema, subretinal (disciform) scarring, and massive subretinal exudation which may give rise to exudative retinal detachment. Vitreous haemorrhage may rarely occur when subretinal blood breaks through into the vitreous cavity. Treatment options include photodynamic therapy, intravitreal steroids, and intravitreal anti-vascular endothelium growth factors.

3. Disc neovascularization (NVD) is highlighted by FA and then shows progressive hyperfluorescence due to leakage of dye. NVD occurs as a response to retinal hypoxia associated with capillary non-perfusion. Important causes are diabetes, venous occlusion, occlusive vasculitis, and radiation retinopathy. Treatment to prevent vitreous haemorrhage involves laser panretinal photocoagulation.

4. Cystoid macular oedema (CMO) has many diverse causes such as retinal vascular disease, intraocular inflammation, and intraocular surgery. Late phase FA shows a 'flower-petal' pattern of hyperfluorescence caused by accumulation of dye within microcystic spaces. In the short term CMO is innocuous but severe long-standing cases may lead to coalescence of the microcystic spaces into larger cavities and subsequent lamellar hole formation resulting in irreversible damage to central vision.

5. Idiopathic juxtafoveolar retinal telangiectasis is a rare congenital or acquired condition that may cause visual loss as a result of ischaemia or leakage, and the formation of hard exudates.

6. Papilloedema is swelling of the optic nerve head secondary to raised intracranial pressure. It is nearly always bilateral although it may be asymmetrical in severity. Severe long-standing papilloedema causes severe visual loss as a result of secondary optic atrophy.

QUESTION 162

What have these conditions in common?

They were all caused by blunt ocular trauma

1. Retinal dialysis is a circumferential tear along the ora serrata caused by traction of the relatively inelastic vitreous gel along the posterior aspect of the vitreous base. Dialyses most frequently develop in the inferotemporal and superonasal quadrants.

2. Commotio retinae (Berlin oedema) has a grey appearance caused by cloudy swelling of the sensory retina.

3. Macular hole formation may be the result of severe commotio retinae and may give rise to retinal detachment.

4. Optic nerve avulsion is rare but devastating.

5. Vitreous base avulsion may accompany a retinal dialysis. It has the appearance of a 'bucket-handle' which comprises a strip of ciliary epithelium, ora serrata, and the immediate post-oral retina into which basal vitreous gel remains inserted.

6. Choroidal rupture, when old, appears as a white crescent of exposed sclera concentric with the optic nerve head.

QUESTION 163

What are these eponymous conditions?

1. Khodadoust line is characterized by the linear pattern of keratic precipitates associated with an area of inflammation at the graft margin. It is indicative of endothelial rejection following penetrating keratoplasty.

2. Salzmann nodular degeneration is secondary to chronic keratitis, especially trachoma. It is characterized by elevated grey or blue-grey, nodular, superficial stromal opacities, located either in scarred cornea or at the edges of transparent cornea.

3. Mooren ulcer is a rare, idiopathic disease characterized by progressive, circumferential, peripheral, stromal ulceration with later central spread. Bilateral disease is present in 30% of cases and is more aggressive than unilateral involvement, which tends to be more slowly progressive and responds better to treatment.

4. Krachmer spots are subepithelial infiltrates, reminiscent of adenoviral infection, on the donor cornea indicative of stromal rejection.

5. Gundersen conjunctival flap can be used to cover a persistent epithelial defect. It is particularly suitable for chronic unilateral cases in which the prognosis for restoration of useful vision is poor.

6. Thygeson superficial punctate keratitis is an uncommon condition characterized by recurrent attacks of ocular irritation caused by coarse, distinct, granular, greyish, elevated subepithelial lesions, often associated with a mild subepithelial haze.

QUESTION 164

Which of these tumours require treatment?

None

1. Melanocytoma is a rare, distinctive, heavily pigmented tumour which is seen most frequently in the optic nerve head. Treatment is not required except in the very rare event of malignant transformation.

2. Astrocytoma is a rare, benign, innocuous tumour. Most are endophytic, protruding into the vitreous, but exophytic, subretinal tumours can occur. Astrocytomas may occasionally be encountered as an incidental solitary lesion in normal individuals but are most frequently seen in patients with tuberous sclerosis.

3. Choroidal naevus is an asymptomatic usually post-equatorial, oval or circular, slate-blue or grey lesion with detectable but not sharp borders. Surface drusen may be present, particularly in the central area of a larger lesion.

4. Cavernous haemangioma is a rare, congenital, unilateral, vascular hamartoma characterized by sessile clusters of saccular aneurysms resembling a 'bunch of grapes'. The vast majority are symptomatic and innocuous.

5. Retinoma (retinocytoma) is a benign variant of retinoblastoma. It is characterized by a smooth, dome-shaped mass, which slowly involutes spontaneously to a calcified mass associated with RPE alteration and chorioretinal atrophy. The final appearance is remarkably similar to that of a retinoblastoma following irradiation.

6. Congenital hamartoma of the RPE is a rare entity, usually incidentally diagnosed in asymptomatic children and young adults. It is characterized by a small, jet-black, nodular lesion, with well-defined margins, which usually appears to involve the full-thickness of the retina. It is typically located immediately adjacent to the foveola.

QUESTION 165

What are the ocular manifestations of these syndromic conditions?

1. Sipple syndrome (multiple endocrine neoplasia type IIB) is an AD condition characterized by multiple neuromas on the tongue, lips, and intestinal mucosa, marfanoid habitus, medullary carcinoma, phaeochromocytoma, and hyperparathyroidism. The main ocular manifestations are eyelid neurofibromas and prominent corneal nerves.

2. Stevens–Johnson syndrome is a mucocutaneous blistering disease that is thought to be either a delayed hypersensitivity response to drugs or to epithelial cell antigens modified by drug exposure. Involvement of mouth and haemorrhagic crusting of the lips is typical. Ocular manifestations include a transient self-limiting papillary conjunctivitis, and severe membranous or pseudomembranous conjunctivitis that may lead to severe scarring and secondary corneal changes.

3. Rendu–Osler–Weber syndrome (hereditary haemorrhagic telangiectasis) is an AD condition characterized by telangiectasis of the skin and mouth, and bleeding from the gut and lungs, which may be lethal. Occasional ocular manifestations are conjunctival telangiectasis and retinal haemorrhages.

4. Parry–Romberg is characterized by progressive facial hemiatrophy. Ocular manifestations include poliosis, enophthalmos, congenital iris hypochromia, and Horner syndrome.

5. Crouzon syndrome is an AD craniosynostosis characterized by a wide cranium, short anteroposterior head diameter, maxillary hypoplasia, and a curved parrot-like nose. Ocular manifestations are shallow obits, V-pattern exotropia, and occasionally optic atrophy.

6. Pierre Robin syndrome is an AR disorder characterized by micrognathia and cleft palate, often associated with glossoptosis and laryngeal displacement. Uveal colobomas are the only ocular manifestation.

QUESTION 166

What are the main ocular manifestations of these systemic conditions?

1. Anaemia causes pallor and atrophic glossitis (atrophy of papillae), if caused by iron deficiency. Retinal changes are usually innocuous and rarely of diagnostic importance. Venous tortuosity is related to the severity of anaemia, but other signs such as haemorrhages, Roth spots and cotton-wool spots usually represent coexisting thrombocytopenia in aplastic anaemia. Optic neuropathy may occur in pernicious anaemia.

2. Giant cell arteritis (GCA) is a granulomatous necrotizing arteritis with a predilection for large and medium-size arteries. Superficial temporal arteritis is characterized by a thickened, tender, inflamed, and nodular artery which cannot be flattened against the skull. Pulsation is initially present, but later ceases – a sign strongly suggestive of GCA. By far the most common ocular manifestation is anterior ischaemic optic neuropathy, which may involve both eyes. Other problems include amaurosis fugax, cotton-wool spots, cilioretinal artery occlusion, central retinal artery occlusion, ocular ischaemic syndrome, and ophthalmoplegia.

3. Acne rosacea is a common, idiopathic, chronic dermatosis involving the sun-exposed skin of the face and upper neck characterized by telangiectasis, papules and pustules, and sebaceous gland hypertrophy. Ocular manifestations include conjunctival hyperaemia, chronic posterior blepharitis, and inferior peripheral corneal vascularization, infiltration, and thinning.

4. Acromegaly is caused by excessive growth hormone secretion by a pituitary acidophil adenoma, during adult life after epiphyseal closure. Clinical features include facial coarseness with thick lips and exaggerated nasal folds, enlargement of the jaw, and enlargement of the head, hands and feet, internal organs, and the tongue. The tumour may press on the optic chasm and cause bilateral hemianopia and optic atrophy. Angioid streaks and see-saw nystagmus of Maddox are rarely seen.

5. Nerofibromatosis-1 is a disorder that primarily affects cell growth of neural tissues. Inheritance is AD with irregular penetrance and variable expressivity. It is characterized by cutaneous neurofibromas which may be discrete or flabby. The main ocular manifestations are Lisch nodules, optic nerve gliomas, and eyelid neurofibromas. Other features include spheno-orbital encephalocele, congenital ectropion uveae, glaucoma, and rarely, retinal astrocytomas.

6. Paget disease is a chronic, progressive metabolic bone disease characterized by excessive and disorganized resorption and formation of bone that causes enlargement of the skull and anterior bowing of the tibias. Occasional ocular features include compressive optic atrophy, proptosis, ophthalmoplegia, and angioid streaks.

QUESTION 167

What vision-threatening complications may these conditions cause?

1. Posterior synechiae may develop in eyes with anterior uveitis that have not received adequate treatment, particularly with mydriatics. If they extend for 360° (seclusio pupillae) impairment will occur of aqueous flow from the posterior to the anterior chamber resulting in angle closure by the peripheral iris and elevation of intraocular pressure.

2. Ischaemic central vein occlusion is characterized on FA by extensive hypofluorescence due to retinal capillary non-perfusion. Visual loss may occur as a result of macular ischaemia and neovascular glaucoma secondary to rubeosis iridis.

3. Contact lens wear is the greatest risk factor for the development of bacterial keratitis. Bacteria in the tear film are normally unable to bind to the corneal epithelium. Following an abrasion and hypoxia bacteria can attach and penetrate the epithelium with the potential to cause infection. Bacteria and amoeba may also be introduced onto the corneal surface by poor lens hygiene or the use of tap water. *P. aeruginosa* and *Acanthamoeba* spp. are significantly more associated with soft contact lens wear.

4. Posterior scleritis on axial CT shows scleral thickening and mild proptosis. Vision may be impaired by exudative retinal detachment, macular oedema, chorioretinal folds, and phthisis bulbi.

5. Severe proptosis may lead to lagophthalmos and exposure keratitis. This in turn may result in epithelial defects, secondary bacterial keratitis, corneal perforation, endophthalmitis and panophthalmitis.

6. High myopia on axial CT shows an enlarged globe and a posterior staphyloma. Complications include maculopathy, which may be wet or dry, and retinal detachment, which may be caused by giant retinal tears.

QUESTION 168

What treatment has been performed?

1. Punctoplasty is used to treat severe punctual stenosis that has not responded to simple dilatation with a Nettleship dilator. The procedure involves removal of the posterior wall of the ampulla.

2. Orbital decompression is performed in patients with thyroid ophthalmopathy and severe proptosis either as primary treatment or when non-invasive methods are ineffective. The procedure should also be considered for optic neuropathy that has not responded to intravenous methylprednisolone.

3. Bandage soft contact lenses may be used to promote epithelial healing in eyes with stromal thinning, by mechanically protecting regenerating corneal epithelium from the constant rubbing by the eyelids.

4. Silicone intubation of the lacrimal passages is often used in conjunction with dacryocystorhinostomy.

5. Drainage of the orbit may be required in patients with orbital cellulitis unresponsive to antibiotics, and in those with orbital or subperiosteal abscess formation.

6. Punctal plugs reduce tear drainage and thereby preserve natural tears and prolong the effect of artificial tear substitutes. They are of greatest value in patients with moderate or severe keratoconjunctivitis sicca that is not controlled by topical treatment.

QUESTION 169

What treatment has been performed and was it successful? (A = before, B = after treatment)

1. Successful laser treatment of central serous retinopathy. Treatment is rarely required because most cases resolve spontaneously. Argon laser photocoagulation to the RPE leak or detachment achieves speedier resolution and lowers the recurrence rate but does not influence the final visual outcome. It is advisable to wait for 4 months before considering treatment of the first attack and 1–2 months for recurrences. Treatment is contraindicated if the leak is near or within the FAZ. Two or three low- to moderate-intensity burns are applied to the leakage site (200 µm, 0.2 sec) to produce mild greying of the RPE. Side-effects include stimulation of CNV, localized scotoma, and enlargement of the laser scar over time. In this case laser therapy has been successful and the detachment has been flattened.

2. Unsuccessful treatment of macular hole. Indications for surgery are full-thickness macular holes of stage 2 and above, associated with a visual acuity worse than 6/9. Best results are achieved with holes of less than one year's duration. However, it is possible to close holes of several years duration with associated improvement in visual acuity and decreased distortion, particularly if internal limiting membrane peeling techniques are used. The technique involves removal of the cortical vitreous, relief of vitreo-macular traction, peeling of the internal limiting membrane, and gas tamponade followed by

strict postoperative face-down positioning. Following successful surgery, visual improvement is achieved in 80–90% of eyes, with a final visual acuity of 6/12 or better in up to 65%. In this case surgery has been unsuccessful and the hole remains open.

QUESTION 170

What are these subtle conditions?

1. Iris naevus and **ectropion uveae.**

2. Iris mammillations are tiny, villiform lesions that are uncommon in normal individuals but occur with increased frequency in patients with congenital ocular melanocytosis, neurofibromatosis-1, Axenfeld–Rieger anomaly, and Peters anomaly.

3. Koeppe nodules at the pupillary border occur in granulomatous anterior uveitis and Fuchs uveitis syndrome.

4. Congenital ocular melanocytosis is characterized by slate-grey episcleral pigmentation. It may occur in isolation or in association with cutaneous involvement (naevus of Ota).

5. Naevus flammeus (port-wine stain) in Sturge–Weber is present at birth and does not blanch with pressure. With age the lesion becomes darker and the overlying skin may become hypertrophic and friable. Ocular manifestations include glaucoma and diffuse choroidal haemangioma.

6. Ashleaf spots are hypopigmented macules in patients with tuberous sclerosis. In infants with sparse pigmentation they are best detected using ultraviolet light (Wood's lamp), under which they fluoresce.

QUESTION 171

Which investigation would be appropriate for these conditions?

1. Magnetic resonance angiography (MRA) is a non-invasive method of imaging the intra- and extracranial carotids and vertebrobasilar circulations to demonstrate stenosis, dissection, occlusion, arteriovenous malformations, and aneurysms. The technique uses the motion sensitivity of MR to visualize blood flow within vessels and does not require contrast. Because the retinal emboli most frequently arise from an atheromatous plaque at the carotid bifurcation and less commonly from the aortic arch, MRA would be the appropriate investigation.

2. B-scan ultrasonography provides two-dimensional topographic information concerning the size, shape, and quality of a lesion as well as its relationship to other structures. Three-dimensional imaging is also available and can be used to measure tumour volume and enhance localization of a radioactive plaque over a tumour. A suspicious choroidal melanocytic lesion can be evaluated with regard to acoustic properties such as hollowness, choroidal excavation, and orbital shadowing. The dimensions of the lesion can also be measured and monitored for evidence of growth.

3. Fluorescein angiography is very valuable in assessing macular pathology in diabetic retinopathy and its suitability for treatment. Eyes with extensive macular non-perfusion (ischaemic maculopathy) do not benefit from treatment, whereas those with focal maculopathy with good macular perfusion are amenable to treatment of focal points of leakage.

4. High frequency ultrasonography utilizes 30–50 MHz and allows high-definition imaging of the anterior segment but only to a depth of 5 mm. It is of particular value in the evaluation of congenital corneal opacification.

5. Magnetic resonance imaging (MR) is the technique of choice for lesions of the intracranial pathways. The optic nerve is best visualized on coronal STIR images in conjunction with coronal and axial T1 fat saturation post-gadolinium images. MR can detect lesions of the intraorbital part of the optic nerve (e.g. neuritis, gliomas) as well as intracranial extension of optic nerve tumours that may cause optic atrophy.

6. Computed tomography is the preferred imaging technique in orbital trauma for the detection and assessment of severity of bony lesions such as fractures. It is also able to detect herniation of extraocular muscles into the maxillary sinus and the presence of surgical emphysema.

QUESTION 172

What are these investigations?

1. Dacryocystography involves injection of radio-opaque dye into the canaliculi and taking magnified images. Failure of dye to reach the nose indicates an anatomical obstruction, the site of which is usually evident. A normal dacryocystogram in the presence of epiphora indicates either functional obstruction or lacrimal pump failure, especially if contrast is retained on the late film.

2. Dacryocystography with subtraction provides a higher quality image.

3. Nuclear lacrimal scintigraphy using technetium-99 is a sophisticated test which assesses tear drainage under more physiological conditions then dacryocystography. Although it does not provide the same detailed anatomical visualization as dacryocystography, it is more sensitive in assessing incomplete blocks, especially in the upper part of the lacrimal system.

4. Stratus OCT is used to analyze optic disc topography and retinal nerve fibre layer thickness in glaucoma.

5. Low frequency B scan ultrasonography can be used for evaluation of orbital pathology, such as childhood periorbital capillary haemangiomas.

6. Corneal topography provides a colour-coded map of the corneal surface. The power in dioptres of the steepest and flattest meridians and their axes are calculated and displayed. Topography can be used to quantify irregular astigmatism, to diagnose early keratoconus and other ectasias, and to evaluate corneal shape after refractive surgery, corneal grafting, and cataract surgery.

QUESTION 173

What treatment has been performed?

1. Exenteration involves removal of the globe and orbital contents in patients with malignant disease that is not suitable for or has not responded to conventional treatment. Examples are lacrimal gland carcinoma, orbital embryonic sarcoma, conjunctival melanoma, and orbital extension of choroidal melanoma.

2. Enucleation involves removal of the globe, mainly in patients with intraocular tumours not suitable for conventional therapy, such as choroidal melanoma and retinoblastoma. It may also be performed in grossly traumatized eyes and in cases of unresponsive bacterial endophthalmitis.

3. Tarsorrhaphy involves the suturing together of the upper and lower eyelids. The procedure may be temporary or permanent, and may be central or lateral, depending on the underlying pathology. Tarsorrhaphy is performed to enhance epithelial healing, and also to protect the epithelium in patients with exposure or neurotrophic keratopathy.

4. Rigid scleral contact lenses may be used to protect the cornea from severe trichiasis, particularly in patients with cicatrizing conjunctival disease.

5. Amniotic grafting may be useful in eyes with persistent unresponsive epithelial defects.

6. Iris suturing may be performed after excision of an iris tumour, provided the defect is not too large.

QUESTION 174

Match the motility defect (1–3) with the scan (A–C)

1 and C

Acoustic neuroma may damage the sixth nerve and give rise to a defect in abduction (**1**). **Coronal MR** with enhancement shows a tumour at the pontomedullary junction (**C**). The first symptom of an acoustic neuroma is hearing loss and the first sign diminished cornea sensitivity. Patients with neurofibromatosis-2 have bilateral acoustic neuromas.

2 and B

Thyroid eye disease has caused left lid lag and left defective elevation due to tethering of the inferior rectus muscle (**2**). **Axial CT** shows bilateral enlargement of the medial and lateral rectus muscles, and right proptosis (**B**).

3 and A

Subdural haematoma with uncal herniation may result from severe skull trauma and cause ipsilateral third nerve palsy (**3**). **Coronal MR** shows the location of the blood and contralateral displacement of the brain and ventricles (**A**).

QUESTION 175

What is the diagnosis?

1. Choroidal metastatic deposits appear as fast-growing, creamy-white, placoid or oval lesions most frequently located at the posterior pole. The deposits are multifocal in about 30% of patients and both eyes are involved in 10–30% of cases. The choroid is by far the most common site for uveal metastases. The most frequent primary sites are the breast in women and the bronchus in men. A choroidal secondary may be the initial presentation of a bronchial carcinoma, whereas a past history of breast cancer is the rule in patients with breast secondaries. Other less common primary sites include the gastrointestinal tract, kidney, and skin melanoma. Patient survival is generally poor, with a median of 8–12 months.

2. Iris melanoma is characterized by a pigmented or non-pigmented nodule at least 3 mm in diameter and 1 mm thick usually located in the inferior half of the iris often associated with surface blood vessels. The tumour usually grows very slowly along the iris surface and may invade the angle. This tumour shows scleral involvement, which is unusual because most tumours are composed of spindle cells, and only about 5% of patients develop metastatic disease.

QUESTION 176

What is the diagnosis?

1. Macular pucker is caused by contraction of an epiretinal membrane that may be idiopathic or secondary to retinal procedures (e.g. cryotherapy), retinal vascular disease, intraocular inflammation, and trauma. Retinal imaging may be helpful in diagnosis. **FA** highlights the vascular tortuosity and may show hyperfluorescence if leakage is present. **OCT** shows a highly reflective (red) layer on the surface of the retina associated with retinal thickening.

2. Retinal pigment epithelial tear may develop at the junction of attached and detached RPE in an eye with a retinal pigment epithelial detachment (PED). **FA** may show choroidal neovascularization during the early phase. The late phase shows relative hypofluorescence over the flap due to the folded over and thickened RPE, with adjacent hyperfluorescence due to the exposed choriocapillaris. **OCT** shows loss of the normal dome-shaped profile of the RPE in the PED, with hyper-reflectivity adjacent to the folded RPE.

QUESTION 177

What is this condition?

Naevus of Ota

Congenital ocular melanocytosis is an uncommon condition characterized by an increase in number, size, and pigmentation of melanocytes. It occurs in the following three clinical settings: ocular melanocytosis involves only the eye; dermal melanocytosis involves only the skin; oculodermal melanocytosis (naevus of Ota) involves both skin and eye. The latter is characterized by episcleral pigmentation and deep bluish hyperpigmentation of facial skin, most frequently in the distribution of the first and second divisions of the trigeminal nerve. Ipsilateral associations include iris hyperchromia (**1**), fundus hyperpigmentation (**2**), trabecular hyperpigmentation (**3**), and occasionally iris mammillations. Uveal melanoma may develop in a minority of white patients.

QUESTION 178

Match the fundus (1–3) with the ERG (A–C)

1 and C

Juvenile Best macular dystrophy stage 2 (vitelliform) develops in infancy or early childhood with a striking round egg-yolk ('sunny side up') macular lesion composed of accumulation of lipofuscin within the RPE (**1**). ERG is normal (**C**) although the EOG is severely subnormal.

2 and A

Congenital retinoschisis is characterized by foveal schisis in all patients and peripheral schisis principally involving the inferior fundus in 50% (**2**). ERG is normal in eyes with isolated foveal schisis, but those with peripheral involvement show a characteristic selective decrease in amplitude of the b-wave compared with the a-wave on scotopic and photopic testing (**A**).

3 and B

Retinitis pigmentosa is characterized by the triad of arteriolar attenuation, mid-peripheral perivascular 'bone spicule' pigmentation, and waxy disc pallor (**3**). ERG shows reduced scotopic rod and combined responses (**B**) during the early stages of the disease. Later the photopic responses become reduced and eventually the ERG becomes extinguished.

QUESTION 179

What are these rare congenital conditions?

1. Peters anomaly is an extremely rare but serious condition which is bilateral in 80% of cases. It is characterized by corneal opacity of variable density associated with a defect in the posterior stroma, Descemet membrane and endothelium with or without iridocorneal or kerato-corneal adhesion. In this case the cornea is very cloudy and ultrasound biomicroscopy (UBM) shows an iris stromal defect, and absence of Descemet membrane and adjacent endothelium.

2. Congenital hereditary endothelial dystrophy is characterized by focal or generalized absence of the endothelium resulting in corneal oedema. UBM shows increased corneal thickness but normal anterior chamber depth.

3. Sclerocornea is characterized by, usually bilateral, variable corneal opacification and vascularization. UBM shows posterior corneal defects with complete disorganization of the anterior chamber.

QUESTION 180

What are these eponymous conditions?

1. Dalen–Fuchs nodules are yellow-white fundus lesions seen in Vogt–Koyanagi–Harada syndrome and sympathetic ophthalmitis. Histologically they consist of granulomas situated between Bruch membrane and the RPE.

2. Bowen disease (intraepidermal carcinoma *in situ*) presents as an isolated red, scaling lesion, which may be misdiagnosed as a patch of psoriasis. Histology shows dysplastic changes throughout the thickness of the epidermis and marked hyperkeratosis. A small proportion of patients subsequently develop invasive squamous cell carcinoma.

3. Flexner–Wintersteiner rosettes are a histological feature of retinoblastoma characterized by a central lumen surrounded by tall columnar cells, the nuclei of which lie away from the lumen.

4. Marcus Gunn jaw-winking syndrome is characterized by congenital ptosis associated with retraction of the upper lid in conjunction with stimulation of the ipsilateral pterygoid muscles such as by opening the mouth.

5. Apert syndrome (acrocephalosyndactyly) is a craniosynostosis characterized by oxycephaly, slight orbital shallowing, midfacial hypoplasia, 'parrotbeak' nose, and antimongoloid slant of the palpebral fissures. Syndactyly of the hands and feet is an important feature.

6. Bielschowsky test is used to diagnose fourth nerve palsy. A positive response is characterized by increased hypertropia on ipsilateral head tilt.

QUESTION 181

What are these inherited conditions?

1. Tyrosinase-negative oculocutaneous (complete) albinism in which the patient is incapable of synthesizing melanin and has white hair and very pale skin, and lack of melanin in all ocular structures. Inheritance is usually **AR**.

2. Dominant aniridia (AN-1) accounts for 66% of cases and has no systemic implications. AN-2 (Miller syndrome) is sporadic and accounts for 33% of cases and carries a 30% risk of Wilm tumour developing during the first 5 years of life. AN-3 (Gillespie syndrome) is AR and accounts for the remainder. It is characterized by mental handicap and cerebellar ataxia.

3. Treacher Collins syndrome is an **AD** mandibulofacial dysostosis characterized by hypoplasia of the maxilla and zygoma, beak-shaped nose, micrognathia, antimongoloid slant of the palpebral apertures as well as colobomas of the lower eyelids and malformed ears.

4. Blepharophimosis syndrome is a rare, **AD** disorder characterized by ptosis with poor levator function, short palpebral apertures, telecanthus, epicanthus inversus, lateral ectropion of lower lids, poorly developed nasal bridge, and hypoplasia of the superior orbital rims.

QUESTION 182

What are the presenting symptoms of these conditions?

1. Macular haemorrhage presents with a sudden positive central scotoma which grossly impairs central vision. The most common cause is a choroidal neovascular membrane.

2. Cellophane maculopathy presents with mild metamorphopsia, although in some patients the condition is asymptomatic. It is caused by a thin layer of epiretinal cells which may give rise to an irregular light reflex or sheen at the posterior pole. The membrane itself is translucent and is best detected by using red-free light.

3. Peripheral chorioretinitis presents with increasing blurred vision due to fine floaters caused by vitritis.

4. Macular hole formation causes a gradual impairment of central vision. Because the central scotoma is small it is frequently noticed by chance when the normal eye is closed.

5. Tractional U-shaped tear causes sudden onset of flashing lights (photopsia), which may be induced by eye movements, and vitreous floaters due to acute posterior vitreous detachment with collapse. Photopsia is probably caused by traction at sites of vitreoretinal adhesions. A solitary floater may be caused by the detached annular attachment of vitreous to the margin of the optic disc (Weiss ring). Cobwebs are caused by condensation of collagen fibres within the collapsed vitreous cortex. A sudden shower of red-coloured or dark spots is usually indicative of vitreous haemorrhage secondary to tearing of a peripheral blood vessel.

6. Retinal detachment causes a visual field defect perceived as a 'black curtain' which is often preceded by symptoms of acute posterior vitreous detachment. A superior detachment will cause an inferior defect and vice-versa. Loss of central vision occurs when the subretinal fluid involves the macula.

QUESTION 183

What multiple signs are present?

1. Bilateral iris colobomas and **left esotropia**.

2. Microphthalmos, persistent pupillary membrane, cataract, and **iris atrophy**.

3. Right microphthalmos and **coloboma of the iris and lens**.

4. Aniridia, intraocular lens implant, and **posterior capsular opacification**.

5. Hard exudates at the posterior pole and **a small juxtapapillary astrocytoma**.

6. Retinal artery macroaneurysm and **subretinal haemorrhage**.

QUESTION 184

Match the diabetic maculopathy (1–3) with the angiogram (A–C)

1 and B

Focal diabetic maculopathy is characterized by well-circumscribed retinal thickening associated with complete or incomplete rings of hard exudates (**1**). **FA** shows late, focal hyperfluorescence due to leakage, and good macular perfusion (**B**).

2 and C

Diffuse diabetic maculopathy is characterized by diffuse retinal thickening and other features of background diabetic retinopathy. Landmarks may be obliterated by severe oedema which may render localization of the fovea impossible (**2**). **FA** shows late diffuse hyperfluorescence which may assume a central flower-petal pattern if CMO is present (**C**).

3 and A

Ischaemic diabetic maculopathy is often associated with preproliferative changes such as cotton-wool spots and deep haemorrhages (**3**). **FA** shows capillary non-perfusion at the fovea and frequently other areas of capillary non-perfusion at the posterior pole and periphery (**A**).

QUESTION 185

What are these rare acquired conditions?

1. Cogan–Reese (iris naevus) syndrome is characterized by either a diffuse naevus which covers the anterior iris or multiple iris nodules. It is one of the three conditions that constitute the iridocorneal endothelial syndrome, the other two being progressive iris atrophy and Chandler syndrome, all of which are unilateral and associated with glaucoma.

2. Phacolytic glaucoma (lens protein glaucoma) is open-angle glaucoma, occurring in association with a hypermature cataract. Trabecular obstruction is caused by high molecular weight lens proteins which have leaked through the intact capsule into the aqueous humour. Lens protein containing macrophages may also contribute to trabecular blockage. The aqueous may manifest floating white particles.

3. Medulloepithelioma (previously known as diktyoma) is a rare, benign or malignant, embryonal neoplasm that arises from the inner layer of the optic cup. It may manifest as an anterior chamber or ciliary body mass containing grey-white opacities consisting of cartilage.

4. Progressive subretinal fibrosis and uveitis syndrome is an idiopathic, chronic bilateral disease characterized by yellow, indistinct subretinal lesions which coalesce into dirty yellow fibrous mounds at the posterior pole and midperiphery.

5. Vitreomacular traction syndrome is difficult to diagnose clinically and is more apparent on OCT. In this condition the vitreous cortex is attached to the fovea and optic disc but detached temporal to the fovea and the area of the papillomacular bundle. This incomplete vitreous separation exerts persistent anterior traction which leads to macular wrinkling and chronic CMO.

6. Retinal vasoproliferative tumour is a gliovascular lesion which can be primary or secondary to intermediate uveitis, ocular trauma, and retinitis pigmentosa. Secondary lesions may be multiple and occasionally bilateral depending on the underlying aetiology. The tumour is characterized by a reddish-yellow, retinal or subretinal mass with telangiectasis most frequently located in the infero-temporal periphery.

QUESTION 186

What are these rare congenital conditions?

1. Posterior lenticonus is usually a sporadic, unilateral condition characterized by a round or conical bulge of the posterior axial zone of the lens into the vitreous which is associated with local thinning or absence of the capsule. With age, the bulge progressively increases in size and the lens cortex may opacify.

2. Persistent pupillary membrane.

3. Microphthalmos with cyst is caused by failure of the optic fissure to close, leading the formation of an orbital cyst that communicated with the eye. The extent of the cystic component is best delineated on CT.

4. Sectoral iris hypochromia, which may occur in Hirschsprung disease.

5. Falciform fold extending from the disc to the ora serrata occurs in persistent posterior fetal vasculature. The eye is typically microphthalmic and retinal detachment is common.

6. Congenital miosis due to absence of pupillary musculature.

Match the clinical signs (1–3) with the histology (A–C)

I and A

Hard drusen appear as small, yellow dots beneath the RPE distributed symmetrically at both posterior poles (**1**). **Histology** shows discrete homogeneous eosinophilic nodular deposits lying between the RPE and the inner collagenous layer of Bruch membrane (**A**).

2 and C

Hard exudates are waxy, yellow lesions with relatively distinct margins often arranged in clumps or rings at the posterior pole (**2**). Their distribution in the two eyes is not symmetrical. **Histology** shows irregular eosinophilic deposits mainly in the outer plexiform layer (**C**).

3 and B

Cotton-wool spots are small, whitish, fluffy superficial lesions which obscure underlying blood vessels. They are composed of accumulations of neuronal debris (**3**). **Histology** shows globular structures (cytoid bodies) in the nerve fibre layer which represent swollen ends of disrupted axons (**B**).

Which of these intraocular tumours may be bilateral?

1. Choroidal melanoma is unilateral. This specimen shows the characteristic 'collar-stud' configu-

ration because the tumour has broken through Bruch membrane.

2. Melanocytoma is unilateral. Histology shows heavily pigmented polyhedral cells with small nuclei.

3. Retinoblastoma may be unilateral or **bilateral**. Heritable tumours are bilateral in 85% of cases, non-heritable tumours are unilateral.

4. Astrocytoma may be unilateral or **bilateral**. Sporadic tumours are unilateral. About 50% of patients with tuberous sclerosis have astrocytomas which are frequently bilateral and multiple. Histology shows proliferation of fibrillary astrocytes with small oval nuclei and cytoplasmic processes.

5. Intraocular lymphoma is usually **bilateral**. Histology of vitreous biopsy shows lymphoma cells with large irregular multilobed nuclei, prominent nucleoli, and scanty cytoplasm.

6. Haemangioblastoma is **bilateral** in 50% of cases. About 50% of patients with solitary tumours and all with multiple tumours have von Hippel–Lindau disease. Histology shows capillary-like vascular channels between large foamy cells.

What treatment has been performed?

1. Prophylactic retinal cryotherapy to multiple breaks in several quadrants. Large areas of cryotherapy may increase the risk of pigment epithelial cell release and subsequent epiretinal membrane formation. Therefore laser is the preferred modality for extensive lesions. For small lesions there is little evidence to suggest an increased risk with cryotherapy as opposed to laser. In most cases the treatment modality is based on the surgeon's preference and experience as well as the availability of instrumentation.

2. Argon laser panretinal photocoagulation for proliferative diabetic retinopathy is aimed at inducing involution of neovascularization and preventing visual loss from vitreous haemorrhage and tractional retinal detachment. Initial treatment involves 1000–2000 burns in a scatter pattern extending from the posterior fundus to cover the peripheral retina in one or more sessions. In eyes with severe NVD, several treatment sessions involving 5000 or more burns may be required.

3. Encircling explants are placed around the entire circumference of the globe to create a 360° buckle and, if necessary, may be augmented by local explants. They are indicated mainly in eyes with extensive retinal detachments associated with multiple breaks in different quadrants.

4. Laser photocoagulation in branch vein occlusion is usually not performed in the absence of vitreous haemorrhage because early treatment does not appear to affect the visual prognosis. If appropriate, scatter laser photocoagulation is performed to the involved sector.

5. Pneumatic retinopexy is an out-patient procedure in which an intravitreal expanding gas bubble is used to seal a retinal break and reattach the retina without scleral buckling. The most frequently used gases are sulphur hexafluoride (SF6) and perfluoropropane (C3F8). Pneumatic retinopexy has the advantage of being relatively quick and minimally invasive.

6. Radial scleral buckling using a sponge explant is mostly used to treat retinal detachment caused by U-tears or posterior breaks. In order to succeed it is vital that the size of the explant is adequate and positioning correct.

QUESTION 190

What are these conditions involving the anterior chamber?

1. Silicone oil migration into the anterior chamber in an eye with an anterior chamber lens implant. Virtually all patients treated with silicone oil injection eventually develop cataract. Silicone-oil induced elevation of intraocular pressure may occur either due to pupil block or trabecular block by emulsified oil.

2. Cortical lens matter in the anterior chamber may occur as a result of incomplete removal of peripheral lens material. Removal is advisable to prevent uveitis.

3. Synchisis scintillans migration into the anterior chamber in an aphakic eye. Synchisis occurs in eyes blinded by severe disease in which there has been previous vitreous haemorrhage. It is characterized by scintillating golden-brown cholesterol crystals freely mobile in liquefied vitreous.

4. Asteroid hyalosis migration into the anterior chamber in an aphakic eye. Asteroid hyalosis is characterized by small, white or yellow-white particles composed of calcium-containing phospholipids suspended like 'stars on a clear night' in a normal vitreous.

5. Vitreous migration into the anterior chamber may occur in eyes with lens subluxation, which may be spontaneous or traumatic, or following inappropriate management of vitreous loss during cataract surgery. Complications of vitreous loss include, anterior uveitis, retinal detachment, and CMO.

6. Hypopyon describes white cells in the inferior part of the anterior chamber that have formed a fluid level. It is a sign of serious disease such as acute anterior uveitis, and microbial endophthalmitis or keratitis. Pseudohypopyon is rare and may be caused by leukaemic infiltration or retinoblastoma involving the anterior segment.

QUESTION 191

What do these angiograms show?

1. Optic disc coloboma is characterized by a bowl-shaped excavation decentred inferiorly so that the inferior neuroretinal rim is thin or absent with normal disc tissue being confined to a small superior wedge. **FA** shows hypofluorescence of the excavation traversed by a few blood vessels.

2. Choroidal naevus is an oval, slate-blue or grey lesion often associated with surface drusen. **FA** shows hypofluorescence of the lesion due to blockage and spotty hyperfluorescence of surface drusen.

3. Cytomegalovirus retinitis is a common ocular opportunistic infection in patients with AIDS. **FA** of fulminating disease shows hypofluorescence due to retinal ischaemia and non-perfusion of a large vessel.

4. Non-ischaemic central retinal vein occlusion is characterized by venous dilatation and tortuosity, extensive flame-shaped haemorrhages, scattered cotton-wool spots, and disc oedema. **FA** shows scattered hypofluorescence of haemorrhages and good capillary perfusion.

5. Normal angiogram.

6. Racemose angioma is a rare congenital malformation characterized by enlarged, tortuous blood vessels that are more numerous than normal with veins and arteries having a similar appearance. **FA** shows filling of the vessels but lack of leakage.

QUESTION 192

What is this disease?

Systemic hypertension

1 Shows hypertensive retinopathy characterized by cotton-wool spots, scattered flame-shaped haemorrhages, and arteriolar attenuation; **2** shows hypertensive retinopathy and exudative retinal detachment in eclampsia; **3** shows a macular star, cotton-wool spots, and mild disc oedema; **4** shows fibrinoid necrosis involving a precapillary arteriole in accelerated hypertension: **5** is an ECG showing left ventricular hypertrophy; **6** shows arteriolosclerosis characterized by a thick vessel with a narrowed lumen.

QUESTION 193

Are these conditions unilateral or bilateral?

1. Xanthelasma is a common usually **bilateral** condition involving the skin near the inner canthi.

2. Brown syndrome is characterized by an elevation defect in adduction. The vast majority of cases are **unilateral**.

3. Lipid keratopathy is characterized by the **unilateral** deposition of white or yellowish deposits in the stroma consisting of cholesterol, fats, and phospholipids. Most causes are associated with previous corneal disease, most frequently viral disciform keratitis.

4. Toxocara granuloma is invariably **unilateral.**

5. Lattice degeneration is a **bilateral** condition characterized by spindle-shaped areas of retinal thinning associated with an arborizing network of white lines. Lattice is present in about 8% of the general population and is found in 40% of eyes with retinal detachment particularly in young myopes.

6. Cicatricial retinopathy of prematurity is a **bilateral** condition characterized by peripheral pigmentation and fibrosis involving the temporal fundus associated with straightening of the vascular arcades.

QUESTION 194

Match the eye (1–3) with the teeth (A–C)

I and A

Sjögren syndrome is an autoimmune disease characterized by keratoconjunctivitis sicca, which gives rise to filamentary keratitis (**1**). A very dry mouth may give rise to dental caries (**A**).

2 and C

Congenital syphilis may give rise to corneal scarring due to interstitial keratitis (**2**). Peg-like incisors (Hutchinson teeth – **C**), a saddle-shaped nasal deformity, and 'sabre' tibias are important stigmata of congenital syphilis.

3 and B

Rieger syndrome is characterized by bilateral iris anomalies such as hypoplasia and holes (**3**), and dental anomalies consisting of small teeth (microdontia) that are fewer than normal (hypodontia) (**B**).

QUESTION 195

Systemic treatment with immunosuppressives or antivirals?

1. Ocular cicatricial pemphigoid is a serious, chronic cicatrizing disease which requires systemic **immunosuppressive** therapy to prevent visual loss. Acute disease is treated with systemic steroids. Treatment of chronic disease may involve dapsone, azathioprine, methotrexate, ciclosporin, and monoclonal antibodies.

2. Mooren ulcer is a rare idiopathic disease characterized by progressive, circumferential, peripheral stromal ulceration. Systemic **immunosuppressive** therapy with ciclosporin should be instituted early in patients with bilateral involvement or advanced unilateral disease.

3. Necrotizing scleritis with inflammation is a painful condition that may give rise to severe scleral thinning with exposure of underlying uvea. It may be associated with underlying systemic disease such as rheumatoid arthritis, Wegener granulomatosis, polyarteritis nodosa, and relapsing polychondritis. **Immunosuppressive** treatment involves steroids, and cytotoxic agents such as cyclophosphamide, azathioprine, and methotrexate.

4. Cytomegalovirus retinitis in patients with AIDS is less common since the advent of 'highly active antiretroviral therapy' (HAART) and its rate of progression has also been reduced. Systemic therapy of retinitis is with **antivirals** such as ganciclovir, valaganciclovir, foscarnet, and cidofovir.

5. Severe retinal vasculitis may occur in sarcoidosis and Behçet syndrome and cause visual loss. Systemic **immunosuppressive** treatment is often required, after any possible underlying infective causes, such as syphilis, has been excluded.

6. Progressive outer retinal necrosis is a rare but devastating necrotizing retinitis, caused by varicella zoster virus that occurs predominantly in patients with AIDS. Early macular involvement is common and the visual prognosis is very poor despite **antiviral** treatment with ganciclovir or foscarnet.

QUESTION 196

Topical treatment with steroids, antivirals or antibiotics?

1. Geographic herpes simplex ulceration is characterized by a large epithelial defect that stains well with fluorescein. Treatment is with **antivirals** such as aciclovir, trifluorothymidine, vidarabine or ganciclovir, which are equally effective.

2. Adenoviral keratitis stage 3 is characterized by anterior stromal infiltrates that may last for months or years before fading. Treatment with topical **steroids** may be considered in patients with poor visual acuity, particularly in an only seeing eye. Steroid therapy does not shorten the natural course of the disease but merely suppresses the corneal inflammation, so that the lesions tend to recur if therapy is discontinued prematurely.

3. A dense central stromal infiltrate associated with an overlying epithelial defect must be assumed to be of infective origin and treated with intensive **antibiotics**. The 'PEDAL' pneumonic is useful in distinguishing non-infectious from infectious corneal

infiltrates. The latter are associated with **P**ain, large **E**pithelial defects, purulent **D**ischarge, **A**nterior chamber reaction (uveitis, hypopyon), and a central **L**ocation.

4. Marginal keratitis is a bacterial hypersensitivity-mediated condition characterized by peripheral subepithelial infiltration separated from the limbus by a clear zone. Spontaneous resolution occurs within 3–4 weeks and mild cases do not require treatment. Large symptomatic lesions respond well to a short course of **steroids**.

5. Phlyctenulosis is a rare condition characterized by an injected limbal nodule that may extend progressively onto the cornea and cause scarring. The condition most frequently affects children and may cause severe photophobia, lacrimation and blepharospasm which can be alleviated by a short course of **steroids**.

6. Vernal limbitis is characterized by gelatinous papillae which may be associated with discrete white spots at their apices (Trantas dots). Treatment is with **steroids**.

QUESTION 197

What are these congenital conditions?

1. Euryblepharon describes horizontal enlargement of the palpebral fissure with associated lateral canthal malposition and lateral ectropion.

2. Eyelid coloboma is an uncommon, unilateral or bilateral, partial or full-thickness eyelid defect. It occurs when eyelid development is incomplete, either due to failure of migration of lid ectoderm to fuse the lid folds, or to mechanical forces such as amniotic bands. Upper lid coloboma occurs at the junction of the middle and inner thirds.

3. Ablepharon-macrostomia syndrome is characterized by deficiency of the anterior lamellae of the eyelids, requiring reconstructive skin grafting. Systemic features are an enlarged fish-like mouth, ear and genital anomalies, and redundant skin.

4. Simple anophthalmos is caused either by complete failure of budding of the optic vesicle or early arrest in its development. It is associated with other abnormalities such as absence of extraocular muscles, a short conjunctival sac, and microblepharon.

5. Anophthalmos with cyst (congenital cystic eyeball) is a condition in which the globe is replaced by a cyst.

6. Epiblepharon is very common in Orientals and should not be confused with the much less common congenital entropion. It is characterized by an extra horizontal fold of skin stretching across the anterior lid margin with the lashes directed vertically, especially in the medial part of the lid.

anterior chamber, and normal intraocular pressure.

4. Bietti crystalline retinal dystrophy is an **AR** condition characterized by numerous, glistening, yellow-white crystals scattered throughout the posterior fundus. With time visual loss occurs due to atrophy of the RPE and choriocapillaris.

5. Dominant drusen (Doyne honeycomb choroiditis, malattia levantinese) is an **AD** condition with full penetrance but variable expressivity characterized by drusen at the posterior pole and peripapillary area. Most patients are asymptomatic until the fourth or fifth decades when they may develop visual loss due to choroidal neovascularization.

6. Central areolar choroidal dystrophy is an **AD** condition characterized by circumscribed RPE atrophy and loss of the choriocapillaris at the posterior pole unassociated with drusen or flecks.

QUESTION 198

What is the mode of inheritance?

1. Microcornea is an **AD**, unilateral or bilateral condition in which the adult corneal diameter is 10 mm or less but other dimensions are normal. The eye has a shallow anterior chamber and is hypermetropic.

2. Ectopia lentis et pupillae is an **AR** disorder characterized by displacement of the pupil and the lens in opposite directions. The pupils are small, slit-like, and dilate poorly.

3. Megalocornea is a **XLR** condition characterized by a corneal diameter of 13 mm or more, a deep

QUESTION 199

Match the corneal ectasia (1–3) with the map (A–C)

1 and A

Keratoconus is a progressive disorder in which the cornea assumes a conical shape secondary to stromal thinning and protrusion (**1**); topography shows irregular astigmatism and a paracentral cone (**A**).

2 and C

Keratoglobus is a very rare condition characterized by generalized corneal thinning and protrusion (**2**); topography shows generalized steepening (**C**).

3 and B

Pellucid marginal degeneration is a rare, progressive, corneal thinning typically involving the peripheral inferior cornea from 4 to 8 o'clock (**3**). The condition is bilateral but frequently asymmetrical; topography shows severe astigmatism and diffuse inferior steepening (**B**).

QUESTION 200

How may these conditions be treated?

1. Congenital delayed lacrimal duct canalization is characterized by epiphora and matting of lashes. **Probing** of the lacrimal system should be delayed until the age of 12–18 months because spontaneous canalization occurs in about 95% of cases. Probing performed within the first 1–2 years of life has a very high success rate, but thereafter the efficacy decreases.

2. A small corneal perforation due to melting may be sealed by the application of cyanoacrylate **glue**. The glue is first applied onto a plastic patch, which is then applied to the involved area, and a bandage contact lens is inserted.

3. A large capillary haemangioma causing mechanical ptosis may be treated by **injection of steroid** (triamcinolone or betamethasone) into the lesion. The tumour usually begins to regress within 2 weeks and, if necessary, further injections may be given after about 2 months.

4. Leaking retinal artery macroaneurysm with macular hard exudates involving the macula requires **laser photocoagulation** to prevent further leakage and visual loss. Laser burns are applied to the lesion itself and surrounding area.

5. Giant retinal tears require **pars plana vitrectomy**, fluid-gas exchange to flatten the retina, injection of heavy liquid to unroll the flap, and either trans-scleral cryotherapy or endolaser photocoagulation to seal the tear.

6. Acute embolic retinal artery occlusion should be treated provided the patient is seen within 48 hours. **Ocular massage** is performed most effectively with a gonioscopic lens for approximately 10 seconds, to obtain cessation of flow, followed by 5 seconds of release. The purpose is to mechanically collapse the arterial lumen and cause prompt changes in arterial flow. If this is not successful, **anterior chamber paracentesis** is performed and intravenous acetazolamide administered. Despite this the results of treatment are often very poor.

Index